The Stress-Proof Brain

Master Your Emotional Response to Stress Using Mindfulness & Neuroplasticity

MELANIE GREENBERG, PhD

New Harbinger Publications, Inc.

Publisher's Note

Distributed in Canada by Raincoast Books

Copyright © 2016 by Melanie Greenberg
New Harbinger Publications, Inc.
5674 Shattuck Avenue
Oakland, CA 94609
www.newharbinger.com

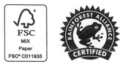

"Practice: Mindfulness of Your Breath" is adapted from MINDSIGHT: THE NEW SCIENCE OF PERSONAL TRANSFORMATION by Daniel J. Siegel, copyright © 2010 by Mind Your Brain, Inc. Used by permission of Bantam Books, an imprint of Random House, a division of Penguin Random House LLC. All rights reserved.

Cover design by Sara Christian; Acquired by Wendy Millstine; Edited by Will DeRooy; Text design by Michele Waters-Kermes and Tracy Carlson

---

Library of Congress Cataloging-in-Publication Data

Names: Greenberg, Melanie, author.
Title: The stress-proof brain : master your emotional response to stress using
    mindfulness and neuroplasticity / Melanie Greenberg.
Description: Oakland, CA : New Harbinger Publications, 2017. | Includes
    bibliographical references.
Identifiers: LCCN 2016036013 (print) | LCCN 2016052428 (ebook) |
    ISBN 9781626252660 (paperback) | ISBN 9781626252677 (pdf e-book) |
    ISBN 9781626252684 (epub) | ISBN 9781626252677 (PDF e-book) |
    ISBN 9781626252684 (ePub)
Subjects: LCSH: Stress (Psychology) | Emotions. | Stress management. | Neuro-
    psychology. | BISAC: SELF-HELP / Stress Management. | PSYCHOLOGY /
    Neuropsychology. | HEALTH & FITNESS / Healthy Living.
Classification: LCC BF575.S75 G6684 2017 (print) | LCC BF575.S75 (ebook) |
    DDC 155.9/042--dc23
LC record available at https://lccn.loc.gov/2016036013

19   18   17

10   9   8   7   6   5   4   3

To Brian and Sydney, who light up my life

Contents

Introduction

You're reading this book because you're stressed. You may be facing stress from some unexpected event or a developmental transition that creates new demands and uncertainty. You may be caring for a new baby, renovating a house, facing a relationship breakup or the loss of a loved one, starting a business, or facing unemployment. Or you may feel chronically stressed on a daily basis by an unhappy relationship, loneliness, weight, a chronic illness, financial struggles, or unrewarding work. Your brain may still be carrying around the emotional burden of childhood trauma or neglect. In addition, you may be dealing with daily frustrations brought about by traffic; bills; home maintenance; demanding family members, bosses, or customers; or an aging body. Whatever the source of your stress, after a while it can make you feel tired, worried, or worn out. But if you understand your brain's hardwired stress response, you can put your brain on a more calm, focused, and positive track. Handling your stress in this way will bring you more happiness and success!

Your Brain Under Stress

When you're stressed out, you feel thrown off balance. Your thoughts race at breakneck speed as you imagine negative consequences or try to come up with quick solutions. Your heart pounds, and your breathing gets shallow as waves of fear emanate from your chest and belly. Your muscles tighten. You feel as if you can't sit still or think straight. You may criticize yourself and regret having gotten into a stressful situation. Eventually, this uncomfortable feeling becomes too much, and you may numb yourself or zone out with food, alcohol, or mindless TV. Or you may drive yourself so hard that you get worn out, become cranky, and find yourself living an unbalanced, unhealthy life.

You may blame and criticize yourself for these unproductive responses to stress, but you shouldn't.

The stress response has been with us for thousands of years. It helped humans survive in the days when we faced threats of starvation and marauding lions and tigers.

The *amygdala*, an almond-shaped structure right in the middle of the brain, evolved specifically to respond to threats. It receives input from the senses and internal organs. When your amygdala determines that a threat is present (for example, you see an angry face or hear a crashing noise), it "sounds the alarm": using hormones and neurotransmitters (chemical messengers), it initiates a cascade of physiological changes that prepare you to either fight or flee. This is why stress can make you feel wound up and irritable or panicky and avoidant.

This stress response is great if you're facing an acute stressor, such as an attacker. Before you even have time to think, your heightened alertness and impulse to fight or escape can save your life. Staying calm and thinking things through at this point would waste valuable seconds.

However, most people very rarely face these types of imminent threats (although the news would have you think otherwise). Far more common are the day-to-day challenges of resolving conflict, getting things done, paying the bills, dating, and taking care of yourself and your family in a changing, challenging world. There are also psychological stressors, such as loneliness, uncertainty, failure, rejection, and threats to your health, security, and livelihood.

In the short term, stress hormones (such as cortisol) energize you, motivate you to overcome obstacles, and help you focus on the problem. Over time, however, the same hormones can lead to anxiety, catastrophic thinking, or inappropriately impulsive action. They can negatively affect your heart, immune system, weight, and even brain functioning. In other words, your brain's automatic stress response can be helpful when you're facing physical danger or an immediate challenge but it's unhelpful when you're facing prolonged difficulties or repeated obstacles. Therefore, in order to meet your long-term goals—to build financial stability, find and maintain a loving relationship, care for a family, own a home, or succeed at a job or business—you need to manage your stress so that it doesn't derail you. You need to learn to master normal life transitions, to overcome unexpected crises and disappointments, and even to avert potential catastrophes. Even if you're already experiencing the negative effects of stress, it's not too late to make a difference. Your brain and body have remarkable self-healing capacities.

You Can Change Your Brain

Your brain has the ability to regenerate and heal itself through a process known as *neuroplasticity*. You can grow new brain neurons; create new, positive, and productive brain pathways; and enlarge the parts of your brain that help you think clearly so that you view life stressors as manageable challenges rather than insurmountable threats. By harnessing the power of your prefrontal cortex, you can calm down your amygdala so that you can respond more mindfully and effectively to stress.

The prefrontal cortex is particularly large and well-developed in humans and is responsible for our amazing thinking and problem-solving capacities. Located just behind your forehead, your prefrontal cortex is like the CEO of your brain. It can simultaneously hold in mind information from your current situation and from your past experience, helping you make informed choices about the best course of action. When you encounter a stressor, information flows from your sensory organs (such as your eyes and ears) to both your amygdala and your prefrontal cortex. However, the pathway to your amygdala is faster, to allow for emergency action under imminent threat. Your prefrontal cortex responds to stress more slowly than your amygdala, because it has to process a lot more information.

Your prefrontal cortex can also rein in your amygdala. It can tell your amygdala to relax—for example, because the snake you think you're seeing is just a stick lying in the path; because change, uncertainty, and loss are a natural part of life; so that you can stay balanced and take better care of yourself for the long haul; or because there are people and resources that can help you with your problems. Or it can tell your amygdala that you can handle a challenging situation because you're going to persevere and work hard until you've learned all the skills you need.

These are some of the strategies used by a well-functioning prefrontal cortex that has solid neural pathways to communicate back and forth with your amygdala and other parts of your brain. When this process works well, your prefrontal cortex takes over, calms down the panic, and helps you deal wisely and strategically with stressors.

So then why are you feeling overwhelmed by stress? Well, it may be for one of the following reasons:

- You have an overactive amygdala.

- There's a problem in communication between your prefrontal cortex and your amygdala.

- Your prefrontal cortex isn't functioning properly.

- Your prefrontal cortex doesn't have the right information from past experience to calm things down.

- You grew up in chaotic circumstances or faced problems that you were helpless to change, such as an addicted, neglectful, or depressed parent; family violence; or poverty.

- As the result of a string of disappointments and failures, you have automatic negative expectations, a feeling that the world isn't safe or supportive, lack of trust in other people to help you, or lack of self-confidence.

Luckily, your brain's neuroplasticity means that you can redirect your thought processes to build more present-focused and hopeful neural pathways and a more interconnected and smoothly functioning brain.

A Program to Build a Stress-Proof Brain

This book will teach you a set of brain-based coping skills to help you reorient your brain so that it can be more resilient to stress. This program is based on the latest research on stress and emotion, the psychological literature on resilience and success under challenging circumstances, and my own experience training psychologists and treating acutely or chronically stressed clients. This program is also grounded in my experience of growing up in a country (South Africa) facing social and economic turmoil, and having to make difficult decisions about my life path and future in the face of considerable uncertainty.

Although stress is a fact of life, you don't have to let it overwhelm you or keep you stuck in ways of thinking and behaving that interfere with your health, happiness, and ability to meet your life goals. You can become the CEO of your own brain, keeping your prefrontal cortex firmly in charge so that it can calm down your amygdala, making you less reactive to stress. This book will help you

- curb unhelpful responses such as avoidance, rumination, and fearful thinking;

- gain clarity and focus;

- restore your sense of control and a growth mind-set;

- use grit and self-compassion to motivate yourself; and

- live a healthy and balanced life in the face of stress.

In today's rapidly changing world, a stress-resilient brain is the best thing you can have for staying focused, fit, connected, and on top of your game. Although you can't erase negative life events and past mistakes, you can take the lessons from these experiences and turn them into fuel for your journey. You can generate inner calm, build healthy lifestyle habits, and facilitate clear thinking to sustain you for the long haul.

How This Book Is Organized

This book is divided into three parts. In part 1, "Understanding Your Stress," you'll learn about your brain and body's stress responses. You'll also learn what type of stressors you're facing and how stress affects your mental and physical health. In part 2, "Calming Your Amygdala," you'll learn to stay grounded in the present moment, even when your amygdala is sounding the alarm bells. You'll also learn to face and calm down difficult emotions, rather than avoiding them. Finally, you'll learn ways to see your stressors as more controllable and use self-compassion to help your amygdala relax. In part 3, "Moving Forward with Your Prefrontal Cortex," you'll learn to be cognitively flexible and to combat worry, perfectionism, and hypervigilance. You'll learn to recruit your brain to positive ends. You'll also learn how to view your stressors as challenges and focus on expanding your coping skills. You'll learn to be grittier in dealing with your stressor and live a healthy, balanced life despite the presence of stress.

PART 1

Understanding Your Stress

CHAPTER 1

Your Brain's Stress Response

Stress is a fact of life, and it's here to stay. Loss, conflict, uncertainty, loneliness, health challenges, competition, deadlines, and financial strain are things we all experience. Your brain's hardwired response to stress, however, is meant to protect you from *immediate physical danger*. Much of our physiological response to stress was laid down through thousands of years of evolution. A programmed stress response helped our ancestors take fast physical action to keep from being eaten by lions or failing to compete for food. In that sense, it was certainly a good thing! Unfortunately, the same programmed stress response isn't too good at helping us deal with modern-day stresses such as paying the bills, dealing with a grumpy boss or a sick family member, and fighting with our loved ones. These situations don't generally call for physical action—they require understanding people's intentions; dealing with failure, loss, or uncertainty; solving logistical problems; or sustaining mental effort. They require us to process lots of information in a short time, juggle competing priorities, and deal with a rapidly changing world. If you're feeling stressed, it may be because your brain is oversensitive to danger. Your brain may be signaling that situations such as those listed above are threats to your survival and readying you for extreme action that isn't necessary or appropriate to your day-to-day challenges (Sapolsky 2004).

The skills you'll learn in this book will help you calm down your brain's automatic stress reaction, along with excess anxiety and anger, so that the more rational parts of your brain have time to get on board and formulate a more mindful response. With repeated practice of the exercises in this book, your brain will learn to manage stress effectively so that life stressors become manageable challenges rather than insurmountable threats. You may even begin to feel some excitement about mastering the challenges you're faced with in life.

But first you have to understand how your brain and body respond to stress. As I say to my clients—many of whom are facing major life events or chronic stressors such as loneliness, relationship stress, illness, caretaking, building a business, or unemployment—"When you name it, you can tame it."

Acute vs. Chronic Stress

As mentioned, your stress response was designed to help you survive immediate threats. When you use a system designed for acute, life-threatening stress over a long period, it can create "wear and tear" on your mind and body. Acute and chronic stress are different mind-body processes with different effects (Sapolsky 2004).

Acute stress is a response to a short-term stressor, such as making a speech, writing an exam, meeting a deadline, or going on a first date. On one hand, this type of stress can create anxiety and psychosomatic symptoms (such as headache and upset stomach). On the other hand, it can make you feel excited and challenged, giving you energy to perform at your best. Mastering an acute stressor can make you feel more confident, skillful, and mature.

Chronic stress is a response to a stressor that continues for more than a couple of hours or days. Some jobs, such as those in law enforcement, can be chronically stressful. Deadlines, unhappy relationships, taking care of family members, and not feeling competent at your job can also be stressful. Chronic stress can have negative effects on your mind and body, particularly if you feel helpless to change your circumstances: If you can't see your way out of the situation despite your best efforts, you're likely to become worried or depressed. Chronic stress that isn't managed properly can lead to fatigue, high blood pressure, and weight gain.

Luckily, you can learn to manage your stress, whether it's acute or chronic. You can even transform feeling stressed into feeling challenged and energized or feeling grounded and self-confident. Although part of your stress response is hardwired and automatic, you can change the way your brain processes and interprets stress. Repeatedly practicing new ways of thinking and behaving can actually change the neural pathways and chemicals in your brain.

Your Brain Possesses Neuroplasticity

Your brain contains billions of neurons, specialized cells that communicate with each other. Over time, any neurons and neural pathways you don't use weaken and wither away, while the ones you use most often become stronger. Your brain also has the ability to grow new neurons from stem cells.

This ability to change allows your brain's structure and wiring to be molded by experience, a quality known as *neuroplasticity*. A famous saying (attributed to neuroscientist Donald Hebb) is "Neurons that fire together, wire together." When a set of neurons gets activated, they become more closely linked, so that the whole sequence is more likely to repeat in reaction to that type of situation in the future. Your thoughts, feelings, and actions can actually change the structure of your brain over time. This explains why your childhood environment can affect your response to stress decades later. It also gives you the potential to change old behaviors that don't help you meet your present-day challenges. You can literally rewire your brain!

How Ted Changed His Automatic Response to Stress

To illustrate what it means to change an automatic stress response, I'll tell you about my client Ted. (Whenever I discuss clients in this book, I've changed names and details to protect confidentiality.)

Ted was raised by a single mother who lived from paycheck to paycheck. After he graduated from high school, he had to take out student loans and work thirty hours a week to pay for college. He earned a business degree and was recruited by a well-known company, at which, thanks to his conscientiousness and work ethic, he was rapidly promoted. When Ted came to see me for therapy, his company was about to be taken over by a conglomerate, so he was facing the possibility of losing his job or being sidelined.

Ted's skills were highly marketable, and he had saved up a lot of money. Yet he was panic-stricken!

Ted worried constantly about never getting another job and ending up homeless. He was scared that his wife would leave him, although in reality she was loving and supportive.

Ted's brain had been conditioned by his childhood stress to see uncertainty and potential loss as highly stressful. His amygdala labeled his job situation as a huge threat and put his brain and body on high alert. His prefrontal cortex was ineffective at calming down his amygdala; it brought in the information about his past experiences of being abandoned by his father and living in poverty, leading him to feel more fearful.

Ted also felt angry at his company's management for not protecting him better. He constantly felt his heart racing and had butterflies in his stomach. He had difficulty thinking clearly.

Ted stopped exercising, and his weight and blood pressure increased. He started feeling depressed.

In therapy, Ted learned to calm down his amygdala and use his prefrontal cortex more effectively. He learned to see his feelings of fear as part of his automatic stress response and not as an accurate indicator of the actual degree of threat he faced. He learned to tolerate fear and find inner calm by using mindfulness skills similar to those you'll learn in this book. Ted also learned to use his prefrontal cortex to view the situation in ways that could calm down his amygdala. He learned to focus on the fact that he'd survived poverty and was now financially comfortable. He realized his wife loved him dearly and wouldn't leave him, even if he was unemployed. He focused on the skills and competencies (such as a great work ethic) that he already had, as well as on the new skills (such as networking) that he could develop and use to manage the situation. He also learned to take a broader view of his life situation and feel proud of his achievements at work and grateful for his loving wife. This focus led to positive feelings that also calmed down the fear. At the end of therapy, Ted not only was better able to handle his current stress but had tools for managing future stressors.

Stress and Your Emotions

Why did Ted feel so much fear and anger at the prospect of losing his job? And why did he feel depressed after a long period of uncertainty? The emotions of fear and anger are created by your body's physiological stress response, combined with your perception of the situation as a threat. As mentioned, when your amygdala perceives a threat, it executes an automatic program to ready your body to fight or flee. That's because your ancestors faced lions and tigers and had to be able to mount a physical response very quickly. So today, when your amygdala perceives a threat, it initiates "fight or flight" mode: sending glucose to your brain for quick thinking, making your heart pump faster, and increasing blood flow to the large muscles of your arms and legs to prepare your body for fighting or fleeing.

Fear and anger are your subjective experience of your brain's "fight or flight" response. Fear is a more acute response, often directed at a specific object or situation (such as the prospect of losing your job). Anxiety is similar to fear, but more diffuse and long-lasting (such as anxiety about what will happen after you lose your job). (In this book, I use the terms "anxiety" and "fear" somewhat interchangeably.) If a stressor continues for a long time or you face a series of stressors, one after the other, you may start to feel depressed. As a mind-body reaction to a situation that you perceive as uncontrollable and overwhelming, depression is like a "freeze" response to stress. We'll discuss this in more detail later.

In the next section, you'll learn about the structures and processes in your brain that determine your response to stress.

Your Brain's Response to Stress

The parts of your brain that shape your emotional and behavioral response to a stressful situation include your amygdala, hypothalamus, hippocampus, and prefrontal cortex. I'll describe each of these brain structures and their functions below. Although we often talk of the amygdala and hippocampus as being single structures, there are actually two parts to each, one half in each hemisphere of your brain.

- **Amygdala**: Your brain's alarm center. It senses threats and other emotionally significant information and initiates the stress response.

- **Hypothalamus**: Your brain's operations manager. It coordinates the release of stress hormones to ready your body for fighting or fleeing.

- **Hippocampus**: Your brain's biographer. It stores and retrieves conscious memories about the current situation as well as previous stressors you've experienced, how you responded, and resulting outcomes. This allows you to learn from past experience and anticipate what's likely to happen.

- **Prefrontal cortex**: Your brain's CEO. It puts together information from your amygdala and hippocampus to create a planned, motivated response to stress. It communicates back and forth with the amygdala to modify your response as the stressor unfolds.

Your Amygdala

Your amygdala is a small (about 0.5 inch) almond-shaped structure that acts as your brain's alarm system. It receives sensory information and decides whether an event is emotionally important. If your amygdala senses a threat, it "rings a mental alarm bell" to tell your hypothalamus to ready your body to respond. Your amygdala does this very rapidly. You may react emotionally to an object or situation before you can even name it. For example, you may jump—before your brain can even think of the word "snake"—when you see a snake-shaped object on a hiking trail.

In terms of stress, your amygdala can hijack your brain away from what you're doing and into emergency mode when you encounter a stressor. If your amygdala sees the stressful situation as a potential threat to your security, status, or well-being, it puts your brain and body on high alert.

Your Hypothalamus

Your hypothalamus is the operations manager of your brain, responsible for initiating and coordinating your hormonal response to stress. When alerted by your amygdala, your hypothalamus releases corticotropin-releasing hormone (CRH). The CRH in turn signals your pituitary gland to secrete adrenocorticotropic hormone (ACTH) into your bloodstream, where it causes your adrenal glands to secrete cortisol. Cortisol circulates through your body, readying your muscles and organs for emergency responding. There's a negative feedback loop for restoring your body to balance: when your levels of circulating cortisol get too high, they signal your hypothalamus to stop releasing CRH, which leads to less cortisol being produced and the system returns to a non-stressed state.

Your Hippocampus

Your hippocampus is a small, seahorse-shaped structure that stores your conscious memories in an organized way. It retrieves memories from the past that may be relevant to your stressor. Your prefrontal cortex accesses these memories so that you can use past experience to inform your response to stress. This means you can avoid trying to cope in ways that didn't work in the past.

When you face a very intense or life-threatening stressor, the resultant surge of stress hormones may cause your hippocampus to go "offline." This means that the event or situation won't be stored in an organized way in your brain. However, it can still affect your behavior in an unconscious way, through your amygdala, by making you more reactive to other stressful situations. For example, if you were bullied when you were a child, your amygdala may react more strongly to criticism from your boss, even though you're not consciously aware of the connection between those events. Your hippocampus also stores memories about your current response to stress. This means that if you cope successfully, your brain will remember it. This will allow you to feel more confident the next time you encounter that type of event.

Your Prefrontal Cortex

Your prefrontal cortex is your brain's executive center. It's like the CEO of your brain, directing the whole operation. Your prefrontal cortex evaluates the demands of the current stressful situation and ties it to your past experience so that you can respond effectively.

Your prefrontal cortex can be your ally in managing your stress. It allows you to solve complex problems, control your impulses, calm down intense emotions, shift your attention, and adapt to new, uncertain, or changing situations. It's the part of your brain that stops you from "losing it" when your preschooler is still not dressed despite umpteen reminders and you're stressed about being late for work. Your prefrontal cortex reminds you of how much you love your kid and want to be a good parent and inhibits the impulse to act like a shrew! This part of your brain helps you study for exams, refrain from having that extra cookie or drink when you're stressed, or stop watching TV so that you can get your work done.

Your prefrontal cortex also connects to your amygdala and hypothalamus to help regulate your emotional response to stress. This part of your brain can help you suppress automatic fearful or angry responses to stressful situations so that you can respond more mindfully and effectively. Your prefrontal cortex is involved in responses such as compassion, shame, and guilt, which modify your amygdala-based reactivity to stress. When you face the stress of public speaking, your prefrontal cortex reminds you of how passionate you feel about the topic that you're speaking about. And when your partner criticizes you, your prefrontal cortex may remind you that your partner is important to you. This calms down your amygdala and eases your stress response so that you can deal more effectively with the stressor.

Now that you know about the brain structures involved in responding to stress, the next step is to understand how your brain initiates a physiological stress response to ready your body for fight or flight.

Your Physiological Response to Stress

Your stress response consists of a cascade of chemicals that travel rapidly through your body, sending messages to your organs and glands, your large muscles, and even your immune system. In this section, you'll learn how your stress response unfolds, beginning with the release of the hormones epinephrine and norepinephrine by your adrenal glands and continuing with the release of cortisol. You'll also learn about how the sympathetic and parasympathetic branches of your nervous system regulate your physiological stress response, switching it off when your brain senses the threat is no longer present. Finally, you'll learn how your parasympathetic nervous system produces a "freeze" response to stressors that you perceive as severe and uncontrollable.

Stress and Your Adrenal Glands

When your amygdala first notices a stressor, it signals your hypothalamus to initiate a lightning-fast chemical response. Your hypothalamus signals your adrenal glands, situated on top of your kidneys, to release the hormones epinephrine (adrenaline) and norepinephrine into your bloodstream to ready your body for fighting or fleeing. Epinephrine rapidly increases your heart rate and rushes blood to your muscles. It opens airways in your lungs to take in oxygen and send it rapidly to your brain for increased alertness; it also spikes your blood sugar level by increasing the production of glucose in your liver. A surge of glucose provides extra energy to your brain and body. Norepinephrine causes a narrowing of your blood vessels, resulting in higher blood pressure.

Do you remember that old ad from the gasoline company Esso (now Exxon Mobil) that boasted their fuel put a "tiger in your tank," giving your car a fuel injection and performance boost? That ad (which is now in the advertising slogan Hall of Fame) describes your adrenal stress response perfectly! Your tank (meaning your brain and body) gets a supercharged surge of adrenaline and glucose. Your heart beats faster, your brain becomes more alert, and you're ready to "go, go, go."

Your adrenal glands' stress response is a rapid and efficient way of preparing for action in the face of an immediate threat. However, if it goes on for a long time, it can be toxic to your body: continuous surges of epinephrine can make you vulnerable to high blood pressure, cardiovascular disease, and heart attack. Luckily, this book will give you tools for managing stress to help keep those things from happening. Next, let's look at the role of cortisol in your stress response.

Stress and Cortisol

If a stressor persists for more than a few minutes, your hypothalamus signals your pituitary gland to release adrenocorticotropic hormone (ACTH). ACTH signals your adrenal glands to release cortisol. Cortisol elevates your blood sugar and stimulates your liver to produce glucose, which is used by your brain to support attention and alertness. It prepares your organs to withstand stress, pain, or injury. Cortisol also suppresses non-emergency functions related to digestion, reproduction, growth, and resistance to disease. If cortisol sticks around for too long, the resultant immune-system suppression makes you more vulnerable to infection. This is why you're more likely to get sick if you're chronically stressed.

As your circulating cortisol levels rise, they send a signal to your body to stop producing more cortisol, so the process is self-regulating; however, chronic stress, trauma, or a series of acute stressors can disrupt this process. Imbalance in levels of cortisol and other stress hormones can cause physiological wear and tear, known as allostatic load (McEwen 1998). Too much allostatic load increases your risk for heart disease, diabetes, obesity, colds and flu, depression, and anxiety.

In some situations, your body may produce less cortisol in response to stress. This can happen in chronic fatigue syndrome. Living a healthy lifestyle and practicing the coping strategies in this book can help you better manage your stresses, whether they're acute or chronic.

Stress and Your Autonomic Nervous System

Once initiated by your amygdala, your stress response is distributed throughout your body by your *autonomic nervous system* (ANS), which consists of nerve cells in your brain and spinal cord. Your ANS has two branches: your *sympathetic nervous system* and your *parasympathetic nervous system*.

Your *sympathetic nervous system* (SNS) acts as your ANS's accelerator. It communicates with your adrenal glands to stimulate the release of epinephrine and norepinephrine, which put your whole body on high alert and ready for action. When the danger is over, your *parasympathetic nervous system* (PNS) acts as a "brake," calming down your system and facilitating a return to a resting state and continuation of non-emergency functions such as sleepiness, appetite, and sex drive (the fun stuff!)

The interplay between these two branches of your ANS supports a balance between at-rest and emergency functions (known as homeostasis). However, if stress is excessive or too prolonged, your ANS can become inflexible—your PNS is unable to put the "brakes" on anxious arousal. If this happens, your brain and body remain on constant high alert.

When your ANS is working well, it's as if you're cruising merrily down the highway—slowing when you need to, stopping at traffic lights, and then moving forward smoothly into the flow of traffic. When the system gets overused and stops working correctly, it's as if you're hurtling through life with faulty brakes, going way too fast, and wearing your engine out.

So far, we've discussed the "fight or flight" component of your acute stress response. This involves the activation of your SNS and its interaction with your PNS. In the next section, you'll learn about the "freeze" component of your stress response, which is initiated by your PNS in response to severe, uncontrollable stress.

Stress and Your Vagus Nerve

Your brain and body are wired to respond to stress with activation and action. But what if "fight or flight" doesn't work? In the case of an airplane crash, a natural disaster, or some other unavoidable threat, continuing to try to fight or run away from the stressor may not only tax your body but increase your suffering. If you can't get away or defend yourself, the only thing left to do is try to numb yourself to the inevitable pain. And your body has a mechanism to do just that: a primitive, parasympathetic "freeze" response that's carried through your body by your vagus nerve. The "freeze" response isn't unique to humans; it occurs in many animal species. Think of the "deer in the headlights" effect.

To illustrate the response of your vagus nerve to severe, over-whelming stress, imagine there's a car hurtling toward you and you don't have time to jump out of the way. After the initial moment of shock, your body's only defense is to shut down and immobilize itself. This response consists of rapid decreases in heart rate and interruptions in breathing that desensitize you to the pain of inescapable danger. You may feel faint, dizzy, or spaced out. If the situation is extreme, you may even lose consciousness.

I experienced a "freeze" response one time when I was in graduate school. I had slept over at my girlfriend's house so that we could study for an exam together. On the morning of the exam, feeling smug and well-prepared, we were driving to school when another car ran a red light and hit us on my side of the car. I must have passed out, because all I remember is a flash of light and then my friend standing next to me calling my name. When I looked around, the door next to me was hanging by a thread! I had to go to the hospital to get checked out and didn't make my exam, but I was otherwise unhurt. My vagus nerve had protected me from the terror of the situation by shutting my brain and body down. Interestingly, I may pay a price for that today, because I sometimes start when traffic slows down suddenly and my husband doesn't begin to brake (or maybe I'm just a backseat driver!).

You may also experience a "freeze" response in relation to normal stressors that aren't life-threatening—for example, some people faint or get dizzy at the sight of blood. If you were abandoned, abused, or neglected as a child, you may feel frozen or immobilized when faced with rejection, loneliness, job loss, or serious financial stress. That's because your brain didn't learn to be resilient! You, as an adult, have to teach it how.

Past experiences of uncontrollability and failure can make you feel overwhelmed, unconfident, and scared to act. The practices in this book will help you train your brain and body to overcome this sense of helplessness so that you can act more effectively to cope with stress. In the next section, you'll learn how stress affects your brain.

Stress and Neurotransmitters

Neurons in your brain communicate with each other by sending and receiving chemical messengers called *neurotransmitters*. Neurotransmitters involved in responding to stress include dopamine, norepinephrine, serotonin, and gamma-aminobutyric acid (GABA).

Stress increases levels of dopamine in your prefrontal cortex. Dopamine is associated with motivation and reward-seeking, and it plays a role in addiction and aggression. Increased dopamine in your prefrontal cortex can have a motivating effect, helping you perform your best. But if you're too stressed out, excess dopamine can make you act more impulsively (without thinking things through).

Stress also leads to an increase in dopamine and norepinephrine in your amygdala, showing that your amygdala is activated by stress and ready to hijack your brain into emergency mode.

Your hippocampus, or memory center, also gets activated by stress, as shown by increased levels of dopamine, serotonin, norepinephrine, and GABA. Your response to stress is affected by past exposure.

Memories stored in your hippocampus add a layer of motivation or emotion to the stressful situation. Remember that your prefrontal cortex integrates information from your hippocampus about your ability to handle this type of situation and communicates with your amygdala to calm down your stress response. Thinking about how well you've coped with similar stressors in the past can help you feel more calm and grounded. I often encourage my clients to think of stressful situations they've survived or mastered so that they can apply the same skills to their current stressors.

On the other hand, memories of past negative outcomes of stressors or of feeling helpless can increase the stress of the current situation. Your amygdala and hippocampus can communicate with each other directly, without going through your prefrontal cortex. This can create a positive feedback loop that increases your overall stress level and makes it more difficult for your prefrontal cortex to calm things down.

Your stress response plays out in your brain and body through neurotransmitters and hormones that affect both your body's reactions and your emotional response to the situation. In the next section, you'll learn about the long-term effects of chronic stress on your mind and body. Learning about the effects of chronic stress may help motivate you to manage your stress before it becomes harmful to your health.

The Effects of Chronic Stress

Over time, stress can affect your brain, your heart, your weight, your resistance to disease, and even your genetic makeup. Ongoing worry and anxiety can exacerbate your stress and not give your body a chance to rest and recover.

Stress and Your Brain

Prolonged or excessive stress interferes with brain function in a few different ways. Stress impairs your brain cells' ability to transport and use glucose (an important source of energy). Without enough glucose, your brain cells are less resilient and more vulnerable to damage. Your hippocampus is particularly vulnerable to the damaging effects of cortisol. Excess cortisol affects your hippocampus's ability to produce new brain cells and repair existing cells. This can negatively affect your ability to learn, your memory, and your mood. Chronic stress and excess cortisol may strengthen connections between your amygdala and hippocampus in a way that predisposes you to a chronic state of emergency preparedness. At the same time, it can weaken the connectivity between these areas and your prefrontal cortex, leading to less regulation of your stress response by the rational parts of your brain. In other words, too much stress can lead your brain to automatically become more reactive, with less ability to calm down your stress response through logical thinking. That's why strategies in this book such as mindfulness, which increases the connectivity between the prefrontal cortex and amygdala, are particularly effective in calming down stress in your brain.

Stress and Your Heart

When your heart experiences repeated surges of epinephrine (due to chronic stress), the lining of your blood vessels can become damaged, raising your risk of hypertension, stroke, and heart attack. Stress can also lead you to engage in unhealthy behaviors that increase your risk of heart disease: You may overindulge in alcohol, smoke, or eat excessively. You may also become hostile and angry. If this describes you, it's time to take a few deep breaths to put the brakes on your "fight, flight, or freeze" response so that your prefrontal cortex has time to calm things down.

Stress and Weight Gain

Cortisol increases your appetite, because food gives you energy for the upcoming "battle." Cortisol also interferes with sleep, and you eat more unhealthy foods when you're tired. Over long periods, chronic stress can increase your blood sugar and causes your body to hang on to excess fat, especially belly fat. Although this effect of stress may have helped our ancestors protect their organs from injury in battle (Epel et al. 2000), it's bad for your health. In fact, the "apple-shaped" body, with a high waist-to-hip ratio, is a risk factor for heart disease, regardless of your weight. So, if you're one of those people who can't stop "emotional eating," or who can't seem to break through a weight plateau even when you reduce your calorie intake, chronic stress could be the reason why. In that case, the stress-reducing strategies in this book may help you naturally lose belly fat (without dieting!).

Stress and Your Immune System

The first studies of stress and the immune system, in the early 1990s, focused on medical students taking exams. It was found that, during exam periods as brief as three days, students experienced a decrease in immune cells that fight tumors and viral infections (Glaser et al. 1993). Hundreds of subsequent studies in the field of psychoneuroimmunology found clear patterns: Stressing people for a few minutes in the laboratory (by way of having them engage in public speaking or mental arithmetic) resulted in an increase in one type of immunity mixed with other signs of immune weakening. However, chronic stress lasting from a few days to months or years seemed to weaken the immune system (Glaser and Kiecolt-Glaser 2005).

Researchers at Carnegie Mellon University measured subjects' levels of stress and then isolated them in hotel rooms (to minimize outside influences) and exposed them to the common cold. Those who were under more stress were more likely to catch colds (Cohen, Tyrrell, and Smith 1991).

When your immune system faces a harmful virus or bacterium (pathogen), it releases chemicals called *inflammatory cytokines* to fight off the attacker. This response, known as *inflammation*, is a normal process that keeps you healthy. Under non-stressful conditions, after the pathogen has been defeated, a feedback loop involving cortisol (mentioned earlier) reduces the inflammatory response, Too much stress seems to make your immune system insensitive to the signaling function of cortisol. This may make you more vulnerable to allergies and asthma or to inflammatory diseases such as diabetes and heart disease.

Stress and Cellular Aging

In a study of the effects of chronic stress on cellular aging, researchers at the University of California looked at mothers who were taking care of kids with autism and chronic diseases. The researchers measured telomeres, a part of your DNA (your genetic material) that controls cellular aging. One way to picture telomeres is to think of a chromosome (a strand of genes) as a shoelace; the telomere is the plastic tip that protects the DNA from damage. Telomeres naturally thin as they age, making DNA vulnerable to fraying.

It turns out that telomeres are highly sensitive to chronic stress. The moms who reported being more stressed had much shorter telomeres—equivalent to at least ten years of extra aging (Epel et al. 2004). However, moms who didn't perceive their lives as highly stressful, even though they had a child with a chronic disability, didn't exhibit the telomere-shortening effect.

In other words, how you view your stress matters! If you can find a way to lighten your load psychologically, your brain and body will be more resistant to stress, and your stressors won't get "under your skin" as much. This book will provide you with an array of psychological tools for managing your stress, as you'll see in the following chapters. But first, let's take a look at how stressed you're feeling.

How Stressed Do You Feel?

Let's take a moment to assess your "perceived stress" or how stressed you feel, regardless of the reason why. When it comes to predicting how stress will affect your long-term health, your feelings of being stressed and out of control are just as important as the actual stressors you face. This is good news, because you can't always choose what you have to deal with in life, but you can change how you feel and think about stress.

PRACTICE: Measuring Your Level of Stress

For each item, circle the number that best represents your answer, where 0 = never, 1 = occasionally or almost never, 2 = sometimes, 3 = fairly often, and 4 = very often.

In the past month, how often have you...

been upset because of an unexpected event or frustration?	0 1 2 3 4
believed that you couldn't control important life outcomes?	0 1 2 3 4
felt "on edge" and "stressed out"?	0 1 2 3 4
believed that things weren't going your way?	0 1 2 3 4
believed that you had more to handle than you could deal with?	0 1 2 3 4
felt irritable and impatient about small things?	0 1 2 3 4
felt your heart racing or butterflies in your stomach?	0 1 2 3 4
been unable to sleep because of your worries?	0 1 2 3 4
felt anxious when you woke up in the morning?	0 1 2 3 4
had difficulty concentrating because of your problems?	0 1 2 3 4

If you circled at least two 2s, 3s, or 4s, you're probably feeling at least moderately stressed. If you circled many 3s or 4s, you're probably under high stress and aren't managing it well on your own. You may want to consult a mental health professional in addition to using the tools in this book.

Final Thoughts

In this chapter, you learned the difference between acute and chronic stress, how your brain processes stress, and how your hypothalamus, your autonomic nervous system, and your vagus nerve control your body's stress response. You learned how communication between your amygdala, your hippocampus, and your prefrontal cortex can modify your stress response. You also learned about some of the damaging effects of chronic stress and elevated cortisol levels. In the next chapter, you'll learn more about the different types of stressors in life, so that you'll be better able to cope with your specific situation.

CHAPTER 2

What Type of Stressor
Are You Facing?

The first step in managing your stress is to understand what type of stressor you're facing. There are many different types of stressors, including developmental transitions, major life events, chronic stressors, daily hassles, trauma, and fallout from negative childhood experiences. You may be facing stress in an important area of your life, such as work, family, parenting, or health. In this chapter, you'll learn about these different types of stressors, the specific challenges they involve, and what research says about their effects. This chapter will help you know why a situation is stressful to you and whether others find it stressful as well. There are also exercises to help you assess your stressors. Comparing your totals at the end of the chapter to determine your primary causes of stress will help you decide which of the strategies we'll discuss later may be most helpful to you.

Developmental Transitions

Developmental transitions are changes at particular stages of your life that require you to adapt to new circumstances. Going to college, buying a house, starting a new job or program of study, getting married, having a baby, and retiring are all developmental transitions. Often bittersweet, these transitions can bring stress and anxiety as well as a sense of meaning or accomplishment. Take a moment now to assess what developmental transitions you may be facing.

PRACTICE: Assessing Your Developmental Transitions

Place a check mark next to all the events that you experienced in the past year that were at least moderately stressful.

_____   moving house or buying a house

_____   pregnancy or having a baby

_____   adopting a child

_____   kids leaving home

_____   starting a new position or getting a promotion

_____   first year of college, starting graduate study, or transferring schools

_____   getting engaged or married

_____   retiring

_____   graduating from college

_____   other life transition (describe): _____

TOTAL: _____

Although most people adapt to developmental transitions without major upheaval and become comfortable with the "new normal" within a few months, some have a harder time. Your genetic makeup may make you less adaptable to change or more prone to anxiety. In addition, factors such as the following can all affect the amount of stress you feel:

- whether you chose the situation

- the other stresses you're facing at the same time

- the resources and support available to you

- unexpected problems or barriers

- how meaningful the situation is

A recent high-school graduate, Jan was going to her dream school in New York City. She had known she wanted to major in international business and done a lot of research to find the right school. She had liked her roommate right away, was getting good grades, and had found a part-time job that left her with enough money to explore museums and trendy neighborhoods on the weekends. Although she missed her old friends, she felt fulfilled and excited by her new life.

Wendy was also just starting college. She had gotten into a big state school in the Midwest, which was her fifth choice, and she was taking science and math courses in hopes of getting into medical school. Her classes were much more difficult than she had expected, and she was beginning to question her chosen career direction. Wendy came from a small town, and she found the campus big and impersonal. She was shy and felt as if she didn't fit in. As a result, she was gloomy and really missed her family and friends back home. She was also struggling financially. This wasn't at all what she had expected, and by mid-semester, she felt unhappy enough to make an appointment at the campus counseling center.

Why was the transition to college so easy for Jan and so tough for Wendy? Several things made the difference:

- **Degree of choice.** Jan got her first choice of college, whereas circumstances dictated which college Wendy would attend.

- **Adaptability.** Jan felt comfortable in a big, new city, whereas Wendy struggled to adapt.

- **Missing old roles or relationships.** Jan wasn't homesick, whereas Wendy missed the familiarity and comfort of home.

- **Match of abilities to challenges.** Jan's academic abilities matched the demands of college, whereas Wendy's didn't.

- **Social support.** Jan quickly bonded with her roommate, whereas Wendy felt isolated.

- **Meaning and fulfillment.** Jan felt fulfilled by her chosen direction, whereas Wendy was unsure whether premed was right for her.

- **Resources.** Jan had enough money to do some fun activities that relieved her stress, whereas Wendy faced financial difficulty.

Compared to Jan's, Wendy's transition to college was less controllable and less meaningful and fulfilling. The new demands exceeded her skill level both socially and academically, and she felt lonely without friends and family to comfort her. Financial problems added to her stress. Wendy's brain labeled the new academic, social, and financial demands and career uncertainty as threats. Her amygdala generated the "fight, flight, or freeze" response that you read about in the last chapter and hijacked her brain into a chronic stress mode that prevented her from enjoying her new life. Jan, on the other hand, didn't experience this amygdala hijack, or, if she did, her prefrontal cortex was able to quickly step in and calm her down or remind her of the positive aspects of the situation.

Are you like Jan, or are you more like Wendy? If you're like Wendy, you may be tempted to criticize yourself for not adjusting to new situations as well as Jan, especially if someone in your life keeps comparing you to a person like Jan! But it's important to take a step back and see that your circumstances are unique and that your feelings of stress may be normal for your temperament and situation. That being said, you bought this book because you'd like to build a more stress-proof brain. Although you may never be a Jan (and you may not even want to be), you can learn coping skills that can help you be the most resilient version of *you*.

For most of us, developmental transitions are a manageable type of stressor: after a while, we learn to adapt to the new situation.

However, for some people, lack of resources, support, skill, or controllability exacerbates the stressfulness of developmental transitions. In the next section, we'll discuss a type of stressor that also involves life change but lacks the potentially positive and fulfilling aspects of developmental transitions.

Major Life Events

Although most people develop the skills to cope with developmental transitions, there's another category of stressful life events involving failure, threat, or loss that may be more challenging. These *major life events* include job loss, divorce, serious illness, and infertility, as well as a loved one's addiction, affair, illness, or death. Major life events generally cause upheaval, stir up anger, fear, or sadness, and require you to devote time and money to coping with them.

Major life events often involve a loss of something tangible, such as money, property, status, position, or opportunity. In addition, your relationships, your routines, or your health may suffer. On a more abstract level, you may lose a sense of certainty about the future, a cherished goal or dream, feelings of safety and security, confidence in yourself, or confidence in others. You may have to deal with the shock of hearing bad news, anxious anticipation of what's going to happen next, unpleasant medical treatments or legal proceedings, or difficult lifestyle changes.

The number of major life events you've recently experienced can affect your resistance to disease, making you vulnerable to colds and flu. Major life events affect your mental health as well. The more major life events you're exposed to, the more likely it is that you'll be diagnosed with depression or an anxiety disorder. Major life events may also make you more reactive to everyday stresses. A stressor such as unemployment, divorce, or the death of a loved one may sensitize your amygdala, making you more reactive to everyday hassles such as traffic and a messy house. That being said, many people are able to cope with major life events without experiencing long-term negative effects.

In the next section, we'll discuss particular types of major life events such as job losses and relationship breakup. These events may seem to represent failure or obstacles to progress in an important life role. They may create fear and uncertainty, or they may challenge you to let go of certain dreams and change your path. The more unresolved and/or recent the events, the more stress they produce. Take a moment now to assess how many major life events you've experienced.

PRACTICE: **Assessing Your Major Life Events**

Place a check mark next to all the events that don't feel completely resolved for you. Put a double check if they occurred during the past year.

_____   the death of a loved one or pet

_____   an unwanted pregnancy or abortion

_____   infertility, miscarriage, or stillbirth

_____   (you or your partner) getting fired from a job or experiencing unemployment

_____   academic failure

_____   being turned down for a promotion, position, or program

_____   (you or a family member) being diagnosed with a serious or chronic health problem

_____   your partner having a physical or emotional affair

_____   the breakup of a romantic relationship

_____   a falling-out with a coworker, supervisor, or close friend

_____   an elderly family member needing care

_____ serious financial or legal problems

_____ a car or bicycle accident

_____ relocation

_____ other major life event (describe): _____

TOTAL: _____

Next, you'll learn about specific types of major life events and typical reactions to them. Of course, your specific life circumstances; your personal qualities, temperament, and financial resources; and your level of social support will affect how stressful these events are for you.

Unemployment or Job Loss

The worker role is an important aspect of identity and status in our society, and losing your job or not being able to find a job can harm your sense of identity and self-worth. In addition, the resultant financial struggles can keep triggering your amygdala, creating a prolonged "fight, flight, or freeze" response. The financial and psychological impact of unemployment affects the whole family; relationship stress is common when one partner is unemployed. Uncertainty, ongoing financial difficulties, and the need to support a stressed-out or depressed partner can create chronic stress for the other partner as well.

Today, more than 20 percent of Americans laid off in the past five years are still unemployed, creating financial and psychological stress. Two groups especially vulnerable to unemployment stress are millennials looking for a first job after college and workers over the age of fifty. If you're unemployed, the contrast between what you expected life to offer you and what you now have may cause your brain to go into "fight, flight, or freeze" mode.

What's the best way to cope with a long period of unemployment? Research studies show that having routines and projects to structure your time, optimism about the possibility of finding a new job, and support from family and friends can help you maintain a sense of normalcy and preserve your self-esteem (McKee-Ryan et al. 2005). Even more important is to find a sense of positive core identity. The trick is to see yourself as worthy or successful in life despite being unemployed. In other words, you find a sense of identity based on your core values or relationships, rather than on events that you can't control, such as finding a high-paying job. For example, you think of yourself as a good parent; a loving partner, friend, or family member; a person of good character; or someone who contributes positively to your community or makes a difference in the world. The strategies you'll learn in this book can help you find an enduring sense of self-worth so that you can better tolerate unemployment and other stressors.

Relationship Breakups

Many of my clients first come to therapy to prevent or cope with the breakup of a close relationship. Generally, the breakup was unwanted and plays into underlying feelings of low self-worth and insecure attachment.

> Becky's parents were part of the hippie generation who came out west to find peace and love. They ended up finding alcohol and drug addiction instead. Her parents split up when Becky was four, and her mother dragged her from commune to commune, leaving her with strangers while she went out and partied. Becky grew up feeling unimportant and unwanted. When Becky came to see me for therapy, she had discovered that her boyfriend of two years wasn't ready for a commitment. She felt abandoned and rejected. Old childhood feelings of loss and low self-worth came flooding back. She found herself obsessing about her ex-boyfriend all the time and going over every aspect of the relationship in her mind,

judging all the things she had done wrong. She didn't want to leave her apartment for fear she would bump into her ex. She felt tired a lot and had headaches, which got worse as she started drinking more.

What was going on in Becky's brain? Her experience of neglect as a child had primed her brain to turn the acute stress of the breakup into chronic stress. Her amygdala and hippocampus created a mutually reinforcing cycle that exacerbated her ongoing stress response. As a result, Becky felt "frozen," stuck in obsessive thinking about her ex and unable to look for new relationships or activities to replace the lost love. Human beings are wired to connect with other people—our brains perceive loss of partnership and rejection as serious stressors.

Chronic Stressors

Chronic stressors are repeated or continuous stressors in important areas of your life. These areas typically include marriage, parenting, work, school, and family relationships. Chronic stressors are usually common but challenging and painful situations, such as being bullied at school or by your boss; having an unhappy marriage; dealing with an ill, addicted, or mentally ill family member; and having a chronic illness. Take a moment now to assess your chronic stressors.

PRACTICE: **Assessing Your Chronic Stressors**

Place a check mark next to all the stressors you experience on a regular basis.

_____ fights with your partner, roommates, or neighbors

_____ financial stress; too much debt

_____ a partner, child, or parent with a mental or serious physical illness

_____   a partner, child, or parent who abuses substances

_____   caring for a child, adult, or pet with serious illness or disability

_____   a high level of stress or demands at your job

_____   academic or achievement difficulties

_____   loneliness

_____   difficulty fulfilling responsibilities because of time, money, or health issues

_____   a lack of support or cooperation from others

_____   negative interactions with friends, family, or coworkers

_____   a noisy, crowded, or uncomfortable living situation

_____   chronic pain, disease, or disability

_____   monotonous work or not feeling valued for your contributions

_____   excessive travel (for example, a long daily commute or weekly travel for work)

_____   chronic dissatisfaction with your weight

_____   an eating disorder

_____   dealing with a difficult ex-partner or blended-family situation

_____   other chronic stressor (describe): _____

TOTAL: _____

Now we'll discuss several of these common chronic stressors.

Caring for a Family Member with a Disability or an Illness

Taking care of a family member with a disability or serious illness is one of the most difficult types of chronic stress. Caregivers often feel frustrated and overwhelmed. They often can't take a break from providing care without having to find a replacement. Perhaps most stressful of all is being the caretaker of an Alzheimer's patient who can't connect with you in a meaningful way. Many studies show this chronically stressed population is susceptible to impaired immunity and inflammation. Seeing your role as meaningful or chosen can be a protective factor, however. For example, choosing to care for someone out of love for the person or because loyalty and compassion are important values for you can buffer you against feeling stressed.

An Unhappy Marriage or Relationship

Having a chronically unhappy marriage or primary relationship can also cause damaging chronic stress. In one study (Troxel et al. 2005), middle-aged women who reported being dissatisfied with their marriage on two separate occasions (about eleven years apart) were three times as likely to have the metabolic syndrome (a syndrome that includes high blood pressure, high blood sugar, excess fat around the waist, and high cholesterol, all of which are risk factors for chronic disease) as those who were dissatisfied on only one of those occasions or satisfied on both.

Interestingly, those wives who were stressed on only one of the two occasions weren't at increased risk of the metabolic syndrome, indicating that chronic stress, rather than acute stress, was the defining factor. In other words, if you experience happy as well as unhappy times in your marriage, or if you repair and resolve your marital conflicts in a timely manner, this may help protect you from the damaging effects of stress.

Work Stress

Work can be a source of life satisfaction and self-esteem, but it can also be a source of great stress. Many workers report working twelve-hour days, not taking lunch breaks, having work-related neck or back pain, or calling in sick because of stress-related health problems. The Whitehall II study (Marmot et al. 1991), a classic large-scale study of thousands of British civil servants, found that workers in lower job grades (with less status, education, and salary) had more job stress than workers in higher grades and were at greater risk for obesity, smoking, hypertension, and heart disease. So, it's not the boss at head office who feels the greatest stress—it's the worker who has to perform and meet deadlines or quotas without having control over schedules or demands. Highly demanding jobs in which the worker has little control over decision-making or resource allocation are the most stressful.

Job stress also depends on the fit of the worker to the position. Some people thrive in a high-stress, busy environment, whereas others feel overwhelmed. However, some situations are stressful for almost anybody, such as feeling as if your job is at risk or as if you can't trust your bosses and colleagues. The following practice will help you assess your job stress.

PRACTICE: How Stressful Is Your Job?

The following items describe some of the most frequent types of job stress. For each type of stress that you're currently experiencing, write a number from 1 (not at all stressful) to 7 (extremely stressful) that best represents how stressful this aspect of your job is to you.

_____ high demands for productivity/performance

_____ insufficient time, equipment, and/or people to do the job

_____ not enough authority or control over decisions

_____ difficult or demanding people

_____ having to be constantly "on duty" without a break

_____ a lack of meaning in your job or the company's mission

_____ work interfering with family life

_____ insufficient training or support to do your job

_____ a hostile or unreasonable boss

_____ a lack of appreciation or reward for your work

_____ a lack of support from coworkers

_____ monotonous or boring work

_____ job insecurity

_____ not feeling fairly treated or compensated

_____ feeling burned out or exhausted

Pay particular attention to any items you gave a 6 or 7. These aspects of your job could be chronically stressing your body, and it may be time to evaluate your options. Depending on your circumstances, you might want to speak up, ask for more resources or training, develop a better attitude, delegate more tasks, let some things go, or look for a different job.

Loneliness

Feeling lonely is stressful for your mind and body. Our ancestors lived in tribes and relied on others to hunt or gather food, raise their young, and fight off predators. Your brain is wired to connect with other people and it interprets loneliness as a chronic stressor, triggering your "fight, flight, or freeze" response.

You can be lonely even in a crowded room if you don't feel cared about or that your needs are important to others. Therefore, loneliness can be assessed in terms of social isolation or just by how lonely you feel. Both types of loneliness seem to damage your health, but feeling lonely may be even worse. A practice at the end of this section will help you assess your loneliness.

Using tools from molecular biology, researchers have been studying the effects of loneliness on people's genes. They've found that genes that promote inflammation are more active in lonely people; in addition, genes that inhibit inflammation are less active in lonely people (Cole et al. 2007). This may explain why loneliness increases your risk for inflammatory conditions, such as asthma and autoimmune diseases.

Some loneliness may be inevitable as we age: friends die or move away, or family members are too busy juggling work and kids to visit or call. You may be more lonely at certain stages of your life, such as when you start college, after you graduate from college, when you have a new baby, after your kids leave home, or after you retire or lose your spouse. These days, many parents shape their lives around their kids' activities, with little time to deepen and invest in their own friendships, resulting in loneliness when their kids move away. But loneliness can also be a subjective feeling that isn't related to any particular life stage. The following exercise may help you decide whether loneliness is a stressor for you.

PRACTICE: How Lonely Are You?

Place a check mark next to all the statements that are true for you.

_____   I don't have people to hang out with or do things with.

_____   When I need help, there's nobody to ask.

_____   I don't have close friends.

_____   I feel shut out or excluded.

_____ I don't feel part of a group or community.

_____ I don't have anyone to talk to.

_____ My relationships are superficial.

_____ I have a hard time making friends.

_____ I don't get invited anywhere.

_____ I feel alone most of the time.

Most people rate half or fewer of such items as true. If you checked more than half the items, loneliness may be a chronic stressor for you.

In this book, you'll learn strategies for coping with loneliness; however, prevention is better than cure. Having a few close, caring relationships with friends, family, or coworkers and being engaged in a community are good for your physical and mental health, especially when you experience major life stress. So it's important to stay in touch with old friends and family, stay connected to your neighbors or colleagues, and look for ways to be a caring, contributing member of your community.

Daily Hassles

Daily hassles are the minor irritations we all experience: The printer jams, or you lose your keys. You get stuck in traffic, or there's nothing to eat in the house. You get a traffic ticket or have to pay late fees. Your partner is grumpy, or your kids don't pick up their stuff. Your dog gets muddy or digs a hole in the yard.

These annoyances can constantly trigger your stress response at low levels, adding up to a lot of frustration and interfering with your goals. Although some people recover quickly from these types of stressors, others become sensitized and have a stronger reaction. Take a moment now to assess your daily hassles.

PRACTICE: Assessing Your Daily Hassles

Place a check mark next to the hassles you experience on a regular basis.

_____ traffic delays; slow or aggressive drivers

_____ costly or time-consuming home or car repairs

_____ computer or equipment problems

_____ regularly misplacing your keys, your wallet, your phone, or other important items

_____ work or household chores piling up

_____ difficult logistics of child care

_____ other people not doing their share

_____ problems with wildlife, rodents, or pets

_____ demands from family members or friends

_____ too many e-mails, too many calls, or too much paperwork

_____ (you or your family members) having frequent colds or flu

_____ other daily hassles (describe): _____

TOTAL: _____

There are many reasons why daily hassles can engage your amygdala's "fight, flight, or freeze" response. First, they may block you from an important goal, and you may see them as unnecessary or due to incompetence. Many times, I've been stuck behind slow drivers on the one-lane roads that take me to work. I have to watch the way I think about these things. If I start thinking *Why is this person going so slowly? Is she clueless?* or *I could've made that traffic light if he had only moved a bit and now, because of him, I'm stuck for another five minutes*, then I've taken a big turn onto the stress highway. I know my clients don't want to see a therapist who's red in the face and muttering about incompetent drivers, to say nothing about the long-term effects on my health!

A second reason why daily hassles can turn into a major source of stress is that when they accumulate, you don't have enough time to recover from one problem before another rears its ugly head. Our brains and bodies are wired for acute stress followed by recovery, not for a barrage of stressors!

I have a great example of stressor accumulation from my own life. Because housing is so expensive in the Bay Area, most people have no choice but to move into houses built in the 1950s in various states of disrepair. In the past few years, I've spent hundreds of hours dealing with broken dishwashers and washing machines, rat droppings and hornets' nests, raccoons and gophers, electricity that goes out in a storm, sewers backing up, broken pipes, leaky toilets, and a landlord we had to take to small-claims court. I now totally understand why some studies of stress find that daily hassles have a more damaging effect on people's health than even major life events experienced in the past year. When there's no time to recover from one problem before the next one hits, your system starts wearing down from the stress. My way of coping with these unavoidable stressors is to write a book about stress. What's yours?

A third reason why daily hassles can turn into major stress is that when you're already stressed by a major life event, you have fewer resources left to deal with the unexpected stuff or the day-to-day turmoil of life. Many high-functioning executives deal skillfully with major crises at work but stress their spouses out with temper tantrums or lack of cooperation. It's as if, when piled on top of work demands, the continual day-to-day problems and logistics of the household send them over the edge.

Another category of stressor that can have a big impact on your health is adverse childhood events (ACEs). Even though these events happened a long time ago, they may have shaped your brain to be more reactive to current stressors.

Adverse Childhood Events (ACEs)

The memory of traumatic events from your childhood can make you more physiologically and psychologically reactive to current stressful events. This is because traumatic events can affect how you interpret the meaning of stressful events and how easily you get triggered into feeling helpless, unsafe, or incompetent.

It's important to understand and respect your own sensitivities when it comes to stress, so that you don't blame yourself for overreacting. Clients often tell me, "Everybody else seems to just get on with it, whereas I feel paralyzed and scared any action I take will make things worse." These clients may have learned from past trauma that there's no escape from a bad situation. Their brains may have learned to respond to stress by freezing because their past attempts to fight or escape were punished or ignored.

One of the largest studies of relationships between childhood trauma and adult functioning (Felitti et al. 1998; Brown et al. 2009) used physical tests and psychological questionnaires to assess seventeen thousand participants. Almost two-thirds of participants reported having experienced at least one ACE. More than one in five participants reported having experienced three or more ACEs.

The more ACEs participants reported, the worse their health. Those who said they had experienced more ACEs were more likely to have heart or liver disease, to smoke, to suffer from alcoholism, to be a victim of domestic violence, or to be diagnosed with major depression.

From this study, it seems that the stress of experiencing multiple ACEs can affect people's health decades later. That's why the powerful stress-management tools in this book are so important. Take a moment now to assess your ACEs.

PRACTICE: **Assessing Your ACEs**

Place a check mark next to all the events you were exposed to prior to the age of eighteen.

_____   physical abuse

_____   sexual abuse

_____   emotional abuse or a narcissistic parent

_____   physical or emotional neglect

_____   a parent with a mental health or substance abuse problem

_____   parental separation or divorce

_____   a seriously ill or injured family member

_____   being adopted

_____   witnessing family violence

_____   the death of a family member or close friend

_____   homelessness or poverty

_____   being bullied (threats, humiliation, deliberate exclusion, and so on)

TOTAL: _____

If your total is three or more check marks, it's particularly important that you learn to manage your stress.

The next category of events we'll discuss is trauma. The words "trauma" and "PTSD" are often associated with military combat, but there are many different types of trauma, as you'll see below.

Trauma

A trauma is an event that involves a threat to life or physical harm to you or your loved ones. This includes many ACEs as well as other kinds of victimization, such as being raped, being assaulted, being in a serious accident, having a life-threatening illness, serving in military combat, or living through a natural disaster. Following a trauma, about 15 percent of people develop full-blown post-traumatic stress disorder (PTSD), and many others experience ongoing symptoms. Symptoms of PTSD include:

- high anxiety

- angry outbursts

- dissociating or "mentally checking out" when stressed

- reliving the traumatic event

- difficulty remembering parts of the event

- a belief that the world is unsafe

- difficulties with intimacy

- nightmares

Some people with PTSD have lower resting cortisol levels than people without PTSD. In healthy people, cortisol is highest in the morning; in people with PTSD, cortisol levels are more constant throughout the day. Their autonomic nervous systems become more rigid, so they have a hard time winding down in the evening. People with PTSD are also more likely to smoke, are at higher risk of heart attack, and are more likely to experience chronic pain. If you think you may have PTSD, consult a mental health professional for an evaluation.

Take a moment now to assess your level of exposure to trauma as an adult.

PRACTICE: Assessing Your Adult Traumas

Place a check mark next to all the following events you've been exposed to as an adult.

_____ rape

_____ the death of a spouse or child

_____ physical violence (toward you or a loved one)

_____ a natural disaster (earthquake, flood, fire, and so on)

_____ being stalked or physically threatened

_____ robbery or burglary

_____ a car accident in which someone was seriously injured or killed

_____ a serious or life-threatening illness, accident, or injury (your own or a loved one's)

_____ military combat

_____ something shocking or gruesome (in real life)

_____ a verbally or emotionally abusive relationship

TOTAL: _____

How Trauma and ACEs Affect Your Stress Response

Trauma and ACEs can disrupt your brain's chemical response to stress. When that happens, your prefrontal cortex can't properly assess for threat and provide accurate feedback to regulate your amygdala. Your amygdala becomes sensitized and prone to label unexpected events, often sensory ones (such as loud noises), as threats, which triggers your stress response too frequently. Events may trigger unprocessed aspects of past trauma: you may feel bodily discomfort without knowing why, or you may experience rage or anxiety that seems out of proportion to the situation. If you're vulnerable to these effects, psychotherapy or practicing mindfulness and other exercises in this book can help you train your brain to respond more calmly to day-to-day stress.

If in the face of stress or major life events you feel overwhelmed, emotionally flooded, unable to think clearly, or scared to act, this isn't necessarily your fault or a sign that there's something wrong with you. It's likely that your brain's stress response has been affected by trauma or multiple ACEs. You have to keep reminding yourself that it's not your fault. And you can train your brain to become more resilient to stress.

This book will help you have a healthier, more organized response to stress. You'll learn that your brain's automatic evaluation of threat may not be accurate—that just because you feel overwhelmed or frozen doesn't mean that you can't learn to calm down and manage the situation effectively. The next practice will help you gain insight into how past trauma or major life events may be influencing your reaction to current stressors.

PRACTICE: **Seeing How Your Stressors Connect**

In a journal or on a separate piece of paper, describe the stressor(s) you're currently facing. Then read the following questions and write down your answers.

- Might your past stressors or trauma be affecting your appraisal of or response to your current situation? Do you see any similarities between these events? Do you see any differences? Are there choices you have now that you didn't have then?

- Is the current situation activating a long-held negative belief, such as *Bad things always happen to me*? If so, what evidence is there that this belief is true or untrue *right now*?

- Are you using behaviors or rules (such as "Don't ask for help" and "Don't show your feelings") that you developed as a result of stressful events in your past? How helpful are these ways of reacting to your current stressors? If they're unhelpful, what alternative strategies could you try?

- Have you had to cope with a series of life stressors? How is this affecting your reaction to the current situation?

- Describe any new insights you have about how past events are affecting your current reactions to stress. Are there any changes you can make right now that would help you be less reactive or cope more effectively?

In this chapter, you've learned about many different types of stressors. The next section will help you decide which of the strategies we'll discuss in other chapters may be most helpful to you.

Dealing with Your Stressor

Different types of stressors may call for different coping strategies. If you've experienced trauma or multiple ACEs, the strategies in part 2 of this book, "Calming Your Amygdala," are likely to be most useful. Mindfulness, facing and accepting your emotions, self-compassion, and understanding what aspects of the situation you *can* control can help you deal with the emotional aftereffects of these events.

If you're dealing with the fallout from a major life event (such as divorce or the death of a loved one), a chronically stressful situation, or a buildup of daily hassles, the strategies in both part 2 and part 3, "Moving On with Your Prefrontal Cortex," are likely to be helpful to you. In addition to understanding and calming down your emotions, you'll need to rebuild. Seeing your stressor as a challenge, overcoming negative thinking, creating positive mental states, and being gritty will help you move forward. By creating healthy routines, you can lay a foundation for stress resilience.

If your stressors are mainly developmental transitions, then you're lucky, because they're more temporary and controllable and have more positive aspects. Humans have an amazing capacity to adapt to new situations, and what's stressful now may no longer be stressful once you learn new skills or have time to get used to the "new normal." The strategies in both part 2 and part 3 are likely to be helpful to you, for the same reasons listed above.

In addition to the type of event, your perceptions and judgments about the situation will affect your physiological stress response. The following practice will help you better understand your stress reaction, irrespective of what type of stressor you're facing. It'll help you gain insight into why you're feeling so stressed and guide you in changing your thinking or taking action to improve the situation. It may also help you put the stressor and your reactions in perspective and deal with your feelings of stress in a proactive manner, rather than avoiding them.

PRACTICE: Understanding What's Stressful for You

Think about a developmental transition, major life event, chronic stress, daily hassle, or trauma that you're currently dealing with. In a journal or on a separate piece of paper, write a paragraph describing the event (or refer to the description you wrote in the previous practice). Identify the most stressful aspect of the event, and explain why it was so stressful.

Then read the following questions and write down your answers:

- How do you feel about this situation? For example, you may have one or more of the following emotions: anger, sadness, confusion, surprise, fear, shame, guilt, happiness. Try to name the specific emotions you're feeling. Are any emotions in conflict with one another?

- What are the actual or potential losses involved in this situation? They may involve relationships, status or security, material things, hopes and dreams, or other types of loss. What negative outcomes do you fear? How likely are these losses or negative outcomes, and which of them are within your control?

- To what extent did you choose this situation? Is there a way for you to accept this situation, even if you didn't choose it? Can you work on accepting those parts of the situation that are out of your control? What can you do to cope with the things you *can* control?

- How well are you meeting the demands of the stressful situation? Are you getting the work done and completing the tasks that you need to? Are you managing your emotions effectively and making healthy choices? Are you communicating and managing your relationships effectively? What skills (such as assertiveness skills or time management skills) might help you cope? How might you begin learning and practicing these skills?

- Are there other stressors that are draining your energy, making you more anxious, or making the situation more complicated? How can you better focus on one thing at a time?

- What type of help or support do you need to deal with the stressor or its emotional impact? For example, do you need practical help, information, resources, or emotional support? Who might be able to provide these for you?

- What personal meaning or positive challenge can you find in this situation? Is there an opportunity for you to stretch yourself and grow as a person, live in accordance with your values, or meet important personal goals?

Your answers to the previous questions can help you figure out how you feel about a particular stressor, why it's stressful for you, and what skills, supports, and resources can help you cope. When you break the stressor down in a logical, stepwise manner, you're using your prefrontal cortex to regulate your amygdala's threat response, rather than just feeling anxious and overwhelmed.

Final Thoughts

In this chapter, you learned about the types of stressors you have. We discussed how stressful events can accumulate or feed each other, making your amygdala more reactive. You learned that your stress response can be disrupted by childhood adversity or trauma and that past events can make you more reactive to present stressors. The practices gave you greater insight into your stressors, how your stressors interact or accumulate, and what attitudes and actions can best help you cope. Now that you understand what types of stressors you have, you can decide whether (a) practicing acceptance and calming your amygdala or (b) using your prefrontal cortex to facilitate positive attitudes and actions (or both) will be most effective for you. In the remainder of this book, you'll learn a variety of tools for stress-proofing your brain.

PART 2

Calming Your Amygdala

CHAPTER 3

Staying Grounded in the Present Moment

In chapters 1 and 2, you learned how your amygdala "hijacks" your brain into an automatic "fight, flight, or freeze" response to stress that involves anxious thoughts, brain chemicals and stress hormones, and waves of emotion. To effectively manage stress, you need to calm down your amygdala's fear and panic. A mindfulness mind-set and skills are the antidote to being swept away or immobilized by stress. Mindfulness is an open, compassionate attitude toward your inner experience that creates a healthy distance between you and your stressful thoughts and feelings, giving you the space to choose how to respond to them. With mindfulness, you learn how to sit peacefully with your thoughts and feelings in the present moment, creating an inner calm to help contain the stress.

If I had to pick just one tool for dealing with stress, I'd choose mindfulness. Its use is supported by a growing neuroscientific literature, demonstrating actual changes to neurons in the amygdala following mindfulness training. Mindfulness-based interventions have gained the attention of therapists, educators, coaches, and even politicians and business leaders. This brain skill can have far-reaching beneficial effects, not only transforming brain neurons but improving immunity, health, life, and relationship satisfaction. Mindfulness has the potential to make not only individuals but even businesses, institutions, and societies more stress-proof.

In this chapter, you'll learn about mindfulness, its history in ancient Buddhist philosophy, and its current use in the West as a widely accepted and effective mind-body practice. You'll learn the qualities of a mindful mind-set and how to train your mind to be more mindful through meditation practice and mind-set change. Read on, and learn why "The Mindful Revolution," as *Time* magazine dubbed it, is the key to managing your stress!

The Roots of Mindfulness

Mindfulness is both a skill and an attitude toward living that originated thousands of years ago as part of Buddhist philosophy. According to the Buddha, mental suffering (or inner stress) occurs because we cling to positive experiences, not wanting them to end, and we strive to avoid pain, sadness, and other negative experiences. This effort to control our mental and bodily experiences is misguided and out of touch with the reality of living. We can never escape loss and suffering, because these are natural parts of life. Our experiences are always changing. Living things wither and die, to be replaced by new living things. The forces of nature are beyond human control.

The Buddha believed that although pain is inevitable, suffering is not. Suffering results from our attempts to cling to pleasure and push away pain. Buddhist teaching describes suffering in terms of being shot by two arrows. The first arrow is the pain and stress that are an inevitable part of being human. These types of stressors, such as aging, illness, and death, are beyond our control. The second arrow is the one we use to shoot ourselves in the foot by reacting to the natural experience of human suffering (or stress) with aversion and protest. It's as if we've become phobic of our own emotions! When we begin to feel stressed, we create mental stories of worry and regret that compound our mental suffering. We get caught up in negative beliefs about ourselves, regrets about the past, or worries about the future, taking us out of the present moment. Or we try to push our feelings of stress away through addictions and avoidance. These strategies just make things worse. As one of my wisest supervisors once said, "The cover-up is worse than the crime!"

The Buddha also believed that if we can understand the nature of suffering and learn to accept pain and loss with compassion (rather than running away from them), our mental suffering will lessen. We may not be able to get rid of the first arrow of inevitable pain and grief, but we can get rid of the second arrow of self-created mental and emotional suffering. By looking at our own inner experiences with a curious, nonjudgmental, and welcoming attitude, we can learn to better tolerate negative states of mind (such as feeling stressed) and relate to these experiences in a more kind, accepting way. Another truth about suffering that the Buddha understood is that our thoughts, feelings, and physical sensations, like all other aspects of life, are transient and constantly changing. When we directly face and accept negative experiences, they'll move through us, rather than getting stuck. The Buddha also believed that living a life of peace, self-discipline, service, and compassion would create an end to suffering on a higher level.

University of Massachusetts Medical School professor emeritus Jon Kabat-Zinn was the visionary who first introduced mindfulness to the Western medical establishment. He reframed the Buddhist concepts using scientific terminology, added some meditation exercises and yoga stretches, and developed an intensive eight-to-ten-week mindfulness-based stress reduction (MBSR) program that included forty minutes of meditation practice each day as homework. He recruited into the program a group of chronic pain patients who weren't responding to regular medical treatment. Incredibly, these participants reported less pain, improved mood, and better mental health from the beginning to end of the program (Kabat-Zinn 1982; Kabat-Zinn, Lipworth, and Burney 1985), and in comparison to a group of patients receiving the clinic's normal care (Kabat-Zinn, Lipworth, and Burney 1985). And thus the Mindful Revolution was born.

Today, mindfulness-based interventions for pain, stress, depression, anxiety, cancer, addiction, and chronic illness are accepted worldwide. The credibility of mindfulness as an intervention for stress and stress-related illness has been enhanced by its strong neuroscientific base. University of Wisconsin professor of psychology and psychiatry Richie Davidson has been instrumental in demonstrating how mindfulness works in the brain and how it can change brain structure and functioning to facilitate stress resilience and mental health. Dr. Davidson's research team used brain imaging technology to study mindfulness in Buddhist monks and novice meditators (Davidson et al. 2003; Lutz et al. 2004). Their findings suggest that "contemplative practices" such as meditation and mindfulness can improve compassion, empathy, kindness, and attention in the brain. These studies powerfully demonstrate neuroplasticity—that even adult brains can change their structure and pathways with repeated practice of new habits. By practicing mindfulness, you can learn to redirect the emotional reactivity of your stress response into more calm, peaceful, and attentive states.

Mindfulness and Your Amygdala

Your feelings of stress result from your amygdala's seeing external experiences or even your own emotions as threats. This is a problem, both because it's impossible to escape many stressful experiences and because it's impossible to stop stress-related emotions from arising.

The location of your amygdala—in the middle of your brain, beneath your cortex—means that it receives information about threats and initiates your stress response very rapidly, sometimes even before the thinking parts of your brain know what's happening. In other words, you can't stop your amygdala from trying to protect you by initiating a stress response when it senses a change in circumstances that could lead to danger, loss, or pain. And you probably wouldn't want it to! Without your amygdala, you might waltz into traffic, stick your hand on a hot stove, or hang out with unsavory characters without realizing the danger. But you do need to manage your amygdala so that it doesn't compound your stress or create unnecessary suffering for you. By using your prefrontal cortex to calm your amygdala when it overreacts, you can avoid the Buddha's second arrow (unnecessary suffering).

Mindfulness skills are the antidote to the amygdala's rapid reactivity. With mindfulness, you can learn to slow things down long enough for the prefrontal cortex to get on board and steer you through the stressful rough waters. Mindfulness also creates a calm, relaxed state of mind that prompts your parasympathetic nervous system to calm down the physiology of the "fight, flight, or freeze" response and return to balance. Mindful states of mind send signals to your body that slow down your breathing and your heart rate. They tell your parasympathetic nervous system that the danger has passed and it can bring the body back to balance. In the next section, you'll learn more about what mindfulness is and how you can practice it to calm down your amygdala.

What Is Mindfulness?

Think of mindfulness as both an attitude toward living and a resilient-brain skill that reduces your amygdala's reactivity. Jon Kabat-Zinn defined mindfulness as a way of paying attention purposefully and with nonjudgmental acceptance to your present-moment experience (1994). When you adopt the stance of mindfulness toward your own experience in the moment, whatever that may be, you open up the space to sit peacefully with and examine your thoughts, feelings, or body sensations, rather than following your amygdala's instructions to run away, be overwhelmed, or react impulsively. You replace fear of your own inner experience with a curious, gentle, welcoming attitude—free of judgment, self-blame, and aversion. The skill of mindfulness allows you to remain grounded in the present moment even when you face difficult stressors, so that your stressful feelings feel more manage-able or less overwhelming.

A mindful state of mind is a deliberate, purposeful, focused way of looking at your experience in the present. Rather than experiencing stress or anxiety on automatic pilot, when you're mindful you look at your feelings of stress from an observer vantage point. You're aware of the stress flowing through your mind and body without feeling totally merged with it. You maintain the awareness that stress is a moving, dynamic state that's flowing through you but that it isn't all that you are. You're more than whatever's happening in your mind and body at the moment. Mindfulness teachers often use the metaphor that you are the sky and your thoughts and feelings are clouds. The clouds float by, but the sky is always there. The sky provides the canvas for the clouds to float on. So you're the sky, and your feelings of stress are the clouds. You can sit out the storm until the sky is clear!

The most common anchor used in teaching mindfulness is your breath. When you get stressed, your breathing becomes faster and more shallow as your sympathetic nervous system readies your body for fighting or fleeing. When the stressful situation is over, your para-sympathetic nervous system begins slowing your breath and heart rate to put the brakes on your stress response. With mindfulness, you deliberately focus on your breath in a way that slows it down, even though this isn't the explicit goal—the goal is just to watch your breath. With mindfulness practice, your breathing becomes slower and more rhythmic, which slows down your heart rate. The parts of your brain responsible for sensing movement and breathing send signals to your amygdala that the threat is over, and the whole system begins to calm down.

The best way to understand how your body reacts to mindfulness is to experience it. The following practice will teach you to focus on your breath in a mindful way. The more often you do these sorts of practices, the more quickly you'll develop an attitude of mindfulness.

PRACTICE: A Simple Breath Awareness Meditation

Here are some instructions for a basic breath awareness meditation. Do this once or twice a day for two weeks, and observe what happens. There's no right or wrong way to do this practice. Try to accept whatever your individual experience is. The goal is not to achieve perfect focus on your breath, but rather to learn how your mind works! It's normal for your mind to wander, but when you catch your mind wandering and deliberately bring it back, you're learning to mindfully control the focus of your attention.

1. Pick a comfortable, quiet place where you won't be disturbed.

2. Sit with your spine upright on a cushion on the floor or a chair. If you use a chair, make sure your feet are touching the ground. Close your eyes, or maintain a soft, unfocused gaze.

3. Begin to notice your breathing. Try to maintain an open and curious attitude. Notice where your breath goes when it enters and leaves your body.

4. Don't try to force or change your breath in any way. It may change naturally as you observe it.

5. If your mind wanders, note what it's doing, and then gently bring your attention back to your breath.

6. Continue observing your breath for eight to ten minutes. At the end of the practice, notice how your mind and body feel, then slowly come back to the room.

As you continue this practice for two weeks, notice if your mind resists the idea of change by creating judgmental thoughts such as *I won't be able to keep it up* or *It won't do any good*. You don't have to believe your judgmental thoughts; just notice them. Try to replace your judgmental attitude with one of curiosity, and keep an open mind so that you don't prematurely limit your experience.

In addition to paying attention in an open, nonjudgmental way, there are other characteristics of a mindful state of mind that create a powerful shift in brain functioning. In the next section, we'll discuss them in detail.

Characteristics of a Mindful State of Mind

Being mindful is more than meditating or focusing on your breath. Rather, it's a state of mind, characterized by the following attributes.

An Observing Stance

Mindfulness doesn't take away your stressful thoughts and feelings, but it changes your relationship to them. It's as if you're an observer who can look at these feelings without getting consumed by them or pushing them away. Thus, being mindful gives you more mental space and freedom. You don't have to be controlled by your stress response; you can redirect your focus, thereby gaining more control over your behavior when stressed.

Slowing Things Down

When your amygdala senses a stressor, it acts very quickly to "hijack" your brain for emergency action. However, not every stressor is an emergency, and successfully dealing with most stressors requires thinking of solutions, tolerating anxiety and uncertainty, and adapting to new situations. These are all functions of your prefrontal cortex, which is slower to receive and process information than your amygdala. Therefore, the first step in being mindful is to slow things down so that you can take a broader view of the situation before reacting. Mindfulness moves your mind out of "acting" mode into "watching" mode, taking away the sense of urgency and giving your mind and body time to get back in sync.

Focusing on the Present Moment

When you practice mindfulness, you focus your attention deliberately and openly on what's happening in the present moment, both within you and around you. You may notice and describe your sensory experience—what you're seeing, hearing, feeling, or smelling right at that moment. Or you may focus on your breath to see what's happening inside and to ground yourself. This awareness of the present helps you stop ruminating about the past or worrying about the future.

Replacing Fear with Curiosity

Mindfulness replaces fear and emotional reactivity with an open, spacious curiosity. What's that thought or feeling that's arising? What does it look like and feel like? Is this something helpful or important that you want to focus on, or is it just an automatic event that you can observe as it passes through you? How does this emotion or experience change and unfold over time?

Openness and Nonjudgment

Nonjudgment is a key part of mindfulness. When your amygdala triggers your stress response, you automatically begin to label the situation or your reactions as a threat that you need to escape. This is the aversion that the Buddha referred to as the second arrow. By observing your judging mind, you can avoid automatically buying into these negative judgments. You can then deliberately redirect your mind back to observing your thoughts and feelings with an open mind. This transforms your experience of stress by taking the terror and panic out of it.

An Attitude of Equanimity

Based on the Buddha's original teachings about non-attachment to pleasure or pain, a mindful attitude is one of peace, balance, and equanimity. To have equanimity means to let go of "needing" things to be a certain way. Equanimity keeps us from getting shot by that second arrow of addictive cravings or feelings of panic and desperation. Everything is impermanent, everything is changing, and many important life outcomes are at least partially out of our control. Therefore, we need to stand firm and not be swept off balance by stress.

"Being" Instead of "Doing"

When you're stressed, your amygdala creates an impetus for action to eliminate the threat so that you can be safe. Finding solutions or learning new skills in a stressful situation requires a goal-oriented mind-set. But your mind and body also need periods of rest and quiet so that you don't get depleted by too much "doing." Mindfulness teaches you how to just "be" in the moment, without any particular goal or outcome and without judging your experience or wanting to be rid of it.

In the next section, you'll learn to deliberately focus on your body or your sensory experience with mindful openness and curiosity.

The "How" of Mindfulness

It sometimes takes weeks or even months of practice to really understand what it means to be mindful. Following are different ways of practicing mindfulness. Try all of them, or find the one that works best for you. Research shows that practicing mindfulness for at least thirty minutes per day can actually shrink your amygdala (Hölzel et al. 2011).

Optimize your environment for practicing mindfulness. You may want to create a "meditation corner" with a comfortable pillow and some pleasant objects for you to focus on. A scented candle, a flower, or a smooth stone can be an anchor for your mindful attention, as I'll describe later in the chapter. Set aside a time every day for mindfulness practice, and put it in your schedule. You can practice mindfulness lying in bed, sitting cross-legged or in a chair, or even while walking, as you'll see below. Find the way that works for you. You don't always have to practice for thirty minutes. Studies show that five to twenty minutes of meditation per day for five weeks creates some of the same brain changes as longer periods of meditation (Moyer et al. 2011) I suggest you start with eight to ten minutes a day of formal practice and then gradually increase the length of your meditations. And so your mindfulness journey begins.

PRACTICE: Mindfulness of Your Breath

This practice is the one I use most frequently with my clients, because it allows you to really feel and connect with your breath and also to feel grounded and solid in your body. It's my adaptation (with permission) of a mindfulness practice used by Daniel Siegel, author of many books and courses on mindfulness and the brain. This version of the instructions is for when you sit upright on the couch. Feel free to adapt the wording if you're lying on the floor or bed.

1. Sit comfortably on the couch with an upright yet relaxed pose. Now close your eyes or maintain a soft gaze. Let your mind and body begin to settle into the practice, noticing what your body feels like.

2. Focus your attention on your feet. Notice all the parts of your feet that are touching the floor. Notice your toes; where your toes join your foot; the middle of your foot; your heel; your ankle; the whole bottom of your foot; the inside and the outside.

3. Let your feet sink into the floor, noticing the support of the earth and feeling it ground you.

4. Begin to notice all the parts of your body that touch the couch— the back of your thighs, your seat, perhaps your back, your arms, and your hands. Let your hands and feet sink into the support of

the couch and floor. Notice how your body feels as you sit, supported by the couch and floor.

5. Begin to notice your breath. Just breathe easily for a few breaths, noticing where your breath goes as you breathe in and as you breathe out. Notice the pause between your in-breath and your out-breath. If your mind wanders—as it probably will, because that's what minds do—just notice where it goes for an instant and then slowly, gently, direct your attention back to your breath. Continue to do this as you begin to notice your breath in your nose, chest, and belly.

6. Slowly, bring your attention to your breath as it enters your nostrils. Notice whether it's hot or cold, light or heavy, and slow or fast. How does it feel? Notice where your breath touches your nostrils as you breathe in and as you breathe out. Continue to notice your breath in your nostrils for a few minutes.

7. Begin to notice your breath in your chest. Notice how your chest moves up and down with your breath like a wave, moving up as you breathe in and down as you breathe out. Just notice your chest as it expands and contracts with your breath. Watch the rhythmic wave in your chest as you breathe in and as you breathe out. Continue watching your chest for a few minutes.

8. Direct your attention downward, toward your belly. You can put your hand on your belly to help you connect with the spot just below your belly button. This spot is at the very core and center of your body. Notice how your belly moves out when you breathe in and how it moves in when you breathe out. There's no need to force or change your breath in any way. And if your mind wanders, bring it back to your belly kindly and gently. As you notice your breath in your belly, notice whether your breath changes or stays the same. Notice the rhythm of your breath in your belly.

9. As you notice your breath in your belly, begin to expand your attention outward toward your whole body. Begin to notice your whole body breathing as a single unit—breathing in and breathing out in a slow, steady rhythm. Notice the waves of breath as they move in and out of your body—filling your nose, the back of your throat, your chest, your ribcage, your belly, and your whole body with fresh, cleansing air. Notice how your breath travels through your body, and see whether it seems to open up any space in the area it touches. Just notice the rhythm of your whole body breathing as one: first the in-breath, then the pause between the breaths, and finally the out-breath. Breathing in and breathing out...

10. Slowly, begin to bring your attention back to the couch, to your hands and feet. Slowly open your eyes and begin to notice the room around you. Take your time, and notice how your body feels now. Is there any difference from when you began the practice?

When my clients do this practice, many report a deep sense of peace, comfort, and calm. Feeling stressed can create tension, tightness, and constriction in your body, particularly in your chest and belly. This practice can help open up space in these areas. A mindful focus creates distance from feelings of stress and generates a sense of peace and well-being.

Your breath is a powerful anchor for your attention, but this isn't the only way to practice mindfulness. You can also use your senses to create a sense of present-moment awareness and inner peace, as you'll see in the next practice.

Mindfulness of Your Senses

When your amygdala sounds the alarm bells, you lose touch with the present moment as your emergency response kicks in. You may feel compelled to "do something" about the stressor or to run away from the overwhelming feelings. By deliberately focusing attention on your senses instead, you move from a "doing," "getting," or "avoiding" mindset to "noticing and describing" what's around you. This helps you feel more present and connected. We connect with the outside world through our senses. When we're mindful of what's around us, we gain awareness that we're part of a larger world of living and inanimate objects. Connecting with your senses can also be a way of what psychologist Rick Hanson (2009) calls taking in the good, or deliberately directing your brain to focus on relaxing or pleasant things in a way that helps calm down your stress response.

Walking in nature is a wonderful way to practice mindfulness of the senses. Being outdoors and close to nature has a calming influence on your brain and body. When you can't get outside, you can still practice mindfulness of your senses, by adjusting the following practice to your situation. You can sit on your deck or in your garden or even look out the window, or you can look at pictures or photographs of nature scenes.

Exciting new research shows that walking outside in green spaces or even looking at nature scenes can increase your mind and body's resilience to stress. A study of college students (Bratman et al. 2015) showed that walking in green campus parkland reduced anxiety and worry more than walking in a busy street and had some cognitive benefits as well. In another study (Van den Berg et al. 2015), students were shown one of two types of pictures: either nature scenes, with trees and empty pathways, or urban scenes, with cars and people. They were then given a stressful math test. Those who had been shown pictures of trees had faster cardiovascular recovery (for example, their heart rate returned to normal more quickly after the test was over) than those who had viewed urban scenes. Measures of vagal tone showed that their parasympathetic nervous systems were better able to put the brakes on their "fight or flight" response.

PRACTICE: Mindfulness of Your Senses in Nature

As you walk or sit in nature, begin to notice your surroundings as a whole, noticing also how you feel in these surroundings. Notice that you're not alone—you're a part of the rhythm and pace of nature.

1. Bring your attention slowly to *what you see*. Notice the colors: the rich browns of the earth, the greens of the trees, or the blues of the sky or water. Are the colors bright or muted? Notice which ones draw your attention. Notice light and shadows, shapes and textures. Which surfaces are smooth, and which are uneven? Which are shiny, and which are dull? Which have sharp angles, and which are rounded? Just notice everything that you see. Now pay particular attention to one object—perhaps a tree or a flower—and notice its color, shape, and texture.

2. Focus on *what you hear*. Perhaps you hear the chirping of birds, the sound of the wind, or a babbling brook. Notice the sounds your feet make as they crunch on the gravel or sink into the earth. Do you hear people's voices? Do you hear a dog barking? Notice the pitch and rhythm of the sounds. Which ones draw you in? Notice how the sounds emerge and then fade away—try to notice the silence between the sounds. Now pick one of these sounds to focus on. Notice its tone, pitch, and rhythm. Notice whether it stays the same or changes.

3. Notice *what you smell*. The smells around you may be sweet or spicy, earthy or fresh, faint or intense. Now pick just one smell to focus on—perhaps the breeze, the earth, or the flowers—and notice everything you can about it.

4. Notice *what you feel*. Notice the temperature of the air. Notice the feeling of the sun or the fresh breeze on your skin. Notice whether the air is moving fast or slow. Notice the feeling of the ground beneath your feet.

5. Notice *how you feel inside your body*. What's it like inside your chest, your back, and your belly? Do you feel any more spacious and calm than when you began this practice? Do you feel any part of you letting go of tension?

6. Notice how your feet feel as you walk. Try to slow the pace of your walking so that you notice each step: Right foot up, moving forward, and then down. Left foot up, moving forward, and then down...

For a short version of this practice, pay attention to just one sense. For example, focus only on what you see, hear, smell, or feel. Or just notice each step you take as you walk, without focusing on your surroundings. You can also do this practice just about anywhere, at any time—not just in nature.

Mindfulness of Objects

Another way to calm your stressed-out brain is to focus on what's around you. If you're feeling stressed while making a presentation, interviewing for a job, taking an exam, or getting ready for an important dinner party, try silently naming three objects in the room and describing their color, shape, and texture as a quick and easy way of moving your mind from "fight, flight, or freeze" mode to "notice and describe" mode.

At home, create a "mindfulness corner" where you keep objects with interesting colors, textures, smells, or sounds. Use it as a sanctuary when you feel stressed, or simply practice mindfulness there daily. Each time you visit your "mindfulness corner," spend a few minutes examining the sensory qualities of each object. Look at it, touch it, smell it, and taste it if appropriate. Things that might work well for this purpose include seashells, smooth stones, scented candles, mints, sprigs of lavender or rosemary, flowers or leaves, lemons, small glass bottles, wooden beads, soft fabric, and hand cream. You can also buy traditional meditation objects such as a mindfulness bell, a Tibetan singing bowl, a small statue of the Buddha, or a Himalayan salt candle. The options are limited only by your budget!

The exercises in this chapter are great ways to learn and practice mindfulness. Yet as we discussed earlier, mindfulness is also a state of mind and a way of living that's larger than any particular practice. Practicing mindfulness teaches you a stress-proof attitude that you can integrate into every aspect of your daily life. And the more you integrate mindfulness into your life, the more opportunity you'll have to calm your amygdala when it starts trying to hijack your brain. In the following section, you'll learn some ways of making mindfulness part of your daily routine.

Integrating Mindfulness into Your Everyday Life

When you're feeling stressed, it's often because you have too much to do and too little time or because you're dealing with an emotionally difficult situation. Stress takes your mind away from the present moment as your amygdala focuses your attention on what will happen if you don't solve the problems or complete the tasks. Your mind may get tired and murky; you may find yourself getting distracted or zoning out instead of focusing on what's most important. You may run around on automatic pilot as your heart races and your breathing shortens in "fight, flight, or freeze" mode.

The following practice is adapted from a practice used by Dr. Elisha Goldstein (Goldstein 2010). Use it to become more mindful from the moment you wake up until you go to bed at night, constantly redirecting your brain back to the present and weakening your amygdala's power to take away your sense of peace and connection with the world.

PRACTICE: Integrating Mindfulness into Your Daily Routine

When you first wake up, instead of jumping out of bed, make time for the STOP practice described here. It'll help you start your day off on a mindful note. Continue to use this practice throughout the day whenever you begin to feel stressed, as a way of grounding yourself when stress begins to creep in.

1. **Stop.** Stop whatever you're doing, and bring your mind back to the present moment.

2. **Take a breath.** Take a few deep breaths to slow down your "fight, flight, or freeze" response.

3. **Observe.** Begin to notice what you're feeling, thinking, and doing. What's going on in your body? Describe any bodily sensations (such as tightness in your throat or shoulders) you become aware of. Is there an emotion word you can use to describe these feelings (such as "angry" or "scared")? Try to stay in the moment with these feelings and "breathe into them": imagine sending your breath into the areas that feel tight, constricted, or activated by these feelings.

4. **Proceed.** When you're feeling sufficiently present and aware, go about your business in a deliberate way. You may want to simply continue what you were doing, but with a more mindful demeanor.

Here are some other ways to integrate mindfulness into your life as you get ready for and go about your day:

- When you observe your morning routine, notice if your mind is already at work or school, worrying or planning how to deal with your daily tasks and challenges. When you notice your amygdala hijacking your thoughts, bring your attention back to the present moment. If you're in the shower, notice the flow, temperature, and sound of the water, the bubbles, and the smell of the soap. When you drink your morning coffee, notice the smell of the coffee beans, the warmth of the cup, and the taste of the first sip. As you eat your breakfast, slow down and pay attention to the sight, smell, and taste of the food and how it feels to chew and swallow.

- Mindfully greet the other members of your household or your pets. Slow down and focus on what they're saying and their nonverbal expressions. Focus on your feelings of love for them. Take time to say good-bye as you leave the house.

- On your way to your destination, notice what your mind is doing. Try leaving the house a little earlier so that you can walk or drive more slowly. Let the things you would normally see as interruptions or obstacles (such as red lights or delays) be reminders to practice mindfulness. If you feel yourself getting angry or impatient with the traffic or long red lights, direct your attention to your breath or focus on the things you see around you—the cars, the people walking by, the trees, the sky, and so on.

As you walk into work or school, drop off your children, or go about your errands, check in with your body and notice any tension. Bring yourself back to the present moment by slowing down and focusing on your breathing, what you see around you, or the feelings in your feet as you walk. Do the STOP practice if you begin to notice bodily tension or negative emotions arising.

- Practice STOP before checking your phone, checking your e-mail, or logging into social media. Set time limits for these tasks, and don't let them sway you into mindless reactivity that distracts you from what's most important.

- Use STOP or breath awareness practices throughout the day. Notice if your muscles are tense, if your breathing is shallow, or if your mind is wandering. Notice if you're feeling reactive, spaced out, or focused and alert. Change your focus by moving or stretching for a few minutes, practicing mindful breathing, or getting some fresh air.

Mindfulness is a skill you learn through repeated practice. It represents a shift in perspective away from constant focus on stressors and amygdala-driven reactivity. It allows your mind and body to rest peacefully and enjoy the moment despite the stress. Stress can be there, but it doesn't have to consume you and take you away from the people you love, getting your work done, looking after your health, and being present in your life. But mindfulness is more than a change in attitude. With regular mindfulness practice and by adopting a mindful attitude toward living, you can actually change the structure of your brain, as you'll see in the next section.

How Mindfulness Calms Down Your Amygdala

Researchers have been studying the effects of mindfulness on the brain and body for more than twenty-five years using sophisticated technologies such as functional magnetic resonance imaging (fMRI) to scan the brain in real time. They have measured effects of mindfulness on depression, anxiety, physiological responses, blood pressure, and resistance to illness. There's now a wide body of evidence showing that mindfulness works to reduce your body and brain's response to stress, taking away some of your amygdala's power to steer you off course.

Mindfulness-based interventions are associated with improved mood, reduced anxiety, better coping when stressed, enhanced emotion regulation, and less physiological reactivity (such as sweating and rapid heartbeat) in response to stressors. A meta-analysis that pooled the results of twenty mindfulness studies concluded that "the consistent and relatively strong level of effect sizes across very different types of sample indicates that mindfulness training might enhance general features of coping with distress and disability in everyday life, as well as under more extraordinary conditions of serious disorder or stress" (Grossman et al. 2003, 39). This meta-analysis showed that mindfulness training reduced disability and improved mood and quality of life in people dealing with a variety of physical illnesses (such as cancer, chronic pain, and heart disease) and mental health issues. Mindfulness interventions have also been shown to reliably reduce anxiety, depression, and stress in healthy people (Chiesa and Serretti 2009; Khoury et al. 2013).

Studies show that mindfulness training can make the amygdala less reactive to stressors. A study by researchers at the University Hospital Zurich (Lutz et al. 2014) focused on whether mindfulness training could affect the brain when subjects viewed pictures designed to trigger emotions. One group of subjects was given mindfulness training, and the other group (the control group) wasn't. Then both groups were shown pictures while their brains were scanned. Subjects were given clues that indicated whether the next picture would be positive, negative, neutral, or unknown (meaning there was a fifty-fifty chance it could be positive or negative). The subjects in the mindfulness group were instructed to use their mindfulness skills (for example, noticing their reactions without judgment) when the clue indicated that an unpleasant or unknown picture was coming. The brain scans showed that, compared to the control group, subjects in the mindfulness group had less activity in the amygdala and in brain regions involved in negative emotion when they anticipated seeing negative or unknown pictures.

Repeated practice of mindfulness over weeks or months may even change the structure of your amygdala. In a study by Harvard Medical School researchers (Hölzel et al. 2011), an eight-week mindfulness course led not only to reduced stress and anxiety but also to changes in the brain: the amount of nerve cells and neural connections shrank in the amygdala but increased in the hippocampus. Neither of these brain changes was found in the control group.

Scientists have pooled data from more than twenty studies (Fox et al. 2014) to show that mindfulness affects at least eight different brain areas associated with self-regulation, memory, focus, motivation, compassion, and resilience. In particular, mindfulness can strengthen your hippocampus, an area that has many cortisol receptors and can be damaged by chronic stress. Your hippocampus can help you mentally process and file away stressful memories so that they're less likely to be triggered later. This suggests that mindfulness can make your brain more resilient to stress.

These research results are exciting, because they prove that you don't have to live in a monastery or on a mountaintop to calm your amygdala and strengthen your hippocampus with mindfulness. Practicing mindfulness over time makes your amygdala less reactive to negative events or uncertainty in your environment and helps your hippocampus process stressful events more effectively.

Final Thoughts

In this chapter, you learned about mindfulness as both a practice and an approach to living that can help you better deal with stress. Mindfulness has its roots in ancient Buddhist philosophy, but it has been adapted for Western use. Being mindful means having an open, accepting, and compassionate attitude toward your own experience in the present moment, whatever that may be. It means allowing, rather than pushing away your inner experience; it means being in the moment, rather than constantly worrying or rushing around. Mindfulness-based interventions have helped reduce people's feelings of stress, lower their blood pressure, and improve their resistance to illness. Mental health professionals use such interventions to treat depression, anxiety, and substance abuse. Mindfulness has also been shown to shrink the amygdala (the brain's alarm center) and protect the hippocampus from being damaged by stress. The mindfulness practices in this chapter can help you reduce your reactivity to stress. Do them as often as you can!

CHAPTER 4

Facing and Accepting Your Emotions

When you get stressed and your amygdala sends you into "fight, flight, or freeze" mode, you may feel fear, panic, or anger. These emotions can be uncomfortable and difficult to deal with. They may make you feel off-kilter and ungrounded. You may feel immobilized and unable to focus or make a decision. Or you may rush around spinning your wheels without making real progress. You may misdirect the emotions by raging at your partner, your kids, or your pets. Or you may feel angry and criticize yourself for not having things under control. Although stress-related emotions can be uncomfortable, they contain valuable information about your goals and important things you need to pay attention to. In this chapter, you'll learn to calm your amygdala by accepting and soothing stress-related emotions so that they can help you manage your stressors rather than derail you.

How Cultural Views of Emotions Can Get in Your Way

There's no course at school about dealing with emotions (although there should be!). Most of us do the best we can, modeling what we learned from our parents, siblings, and peers. You may have been raised to "stay strong" and not show, express, or even experience any negative emotions (except perhaps anger). So when emotions arise, you shove them right back down and out of awareness, without acknowledging them or becoming aware of how they affect your behavior. You may immediately try to fix things, despite lacking key pieces of information about the situation. If you disregard how you feel, you may just accept the stress rather than dealing with it or you may make choices you later regret.

Shoving your emotions down doesn't make them go away. They eventually reappear, often with greater intensity, making them more difficult to manage than they were in the first place. Your amygdala was designed to sound the alarm bells and remind you of a situation that could have a negative or otherwise emotionally significant outcome. And it'll keep doing so until it gets you to listen!

I've heard many clients say they're scared to let themselves feel their emotions in case the emotions "don't stop" or lead them to lose control. These fears are generally unfounded. Emotions are passing mental and bodily events, and if you can acknowledge them without shoving them down or letting them sweep you away, they'll begin to pass.

But how do you *feel* your emotions without *identifying* with them? Mindfulness-based practices can help you learn to direct your attention toward or away from your emotions in a flexible way. Mentally imagining yourself in an anchored or grounded state can also help you tolerate strong negative emotions or bring you back from a state of panic. Keeping a diary about your experiences of stress can give voice to the emotions you feel while creating some structure and containment. The strategies we'll discuss next build on these principles.

Grounding Strategies

Grounding strategies are things you can do to help you feel solid, soothed, and connected with your surroundings. They involve deliberately directing your attention to some aspect of your experience that's not threatening. You can deliberately move your body or focus on your body's position in space; focus on your sense of touch, taste, smell, or sound; or do an activity that engages your logical mind or helps you express yourself. Other strategies involve imagining yourself in an anchored state, connected to the earth. Grounding takes you out of "fight, flight, or freeze" mode and gives your amygdala time to calm down. These strategies are good for people who have a hard time staying mindful.

There's another benefit to some of the grounding strategies. Negative emotions mainly involve the right hemisphere of your brain. Moving your body or doing a verbal, logical, or organizational task deliberately engages the left hemisphere of your brain. We think best when we're using our whole brain. If we only use one part of our brain, we may be missing some key information about the situation or about the way we feel.

PRACTICES: Grounding Yourself When You Feel Stressed

The following grounding strategies can help you feel calm when stress overwhelms you and break the hold that "fight, flight, or freeze" has on your mind and body. Experiment and then choose the strategies that work best for you. With practice, these strategies will become more effective and easier to carry out. Use your feelings of stress and being overwhelmed as clues to remind you to ground yourself. Soon, you'll feel calmer and more present—able to contain the difficult emotion.

- Imagine a golden cord (or stream of light) growing downward from the base of your spine—through the floorboards, through the earth beneath the floor, to the molten center of the earth. Imagine your cord being tethered to the center of the earth with a big anchor. Feel the connection between your body and the earth. As you breathe in and out, imagine your breath traveling up and down the cord, connecting you to the earth.

- Take off your shoes and walk slowly around the room, feeling the connection between your feet and the carpet with each step. Feel your toes, your sole, and your heel connecting with the carpet.

- Imagine yourself as a big tree. Stretch your arms up to the sky and imagine the branches and leaves. Dig your feet into the floor and imagine them growing roots.

- Rock from one foot to the other. As you rock, notice your toes, the pad of your foot, middle of your foot, the sides of your foot, the top of your foot, your heel, your ankle, your calf, your lower leg, and your upper leg.

- Describe three things in the room in terms of their sensory qualities (color, shape, texture, size, smell, and so on).

- Shake your body. Begin by wiggling your toes, then your ankles, your lower legs, and your upper legs. Then do the same thing with your arms, hands, and fingers.

- Breathe in for a count of four, hold your breath for a count of four, breathe out for a count of four, and then pause for a count of four. Try to slow your breath down each time. Try to move your belly out with each in-breath and deflate it with each out-breath.

- Imagine being in a peaceful place, close to nature. Visualize yourself at the beach, overlooking the bay, in the forest, on a hiking trail, or in a park or garden.

- Drink a cup of tea slowly. First feel the warmth of the cup. Then smell the aroma. Notice the color and texture of the tea. Take a small sip and swirl it around in your mouth. Now swallow. Notice the taste and feeling of the tea as it flows down your throat.

- Smell some lavender, or suck on a peppermint.

- Draw, paint, or color a pattern (mandala, flowers, abstract art, and so on). (You can buy coloring books for adults at many bookstores and online.)

- Pat or hug an animal, or hold your dog or cat on your lap. Look at the animal's face, notice her breathing, and feel her warmth.

- Do a small organizational task.

- Take a warm bath or shower, or cuddle in a blanket and warm socks.

- Listen to soothing music, or read poetry.

- Put an ice pack under your neck, or place a cold cloth on your forehead.

- Do a jigsaw puzzle.

- Go for a walk in your neighborhood or somewhere you can be close to nature.

- Walk barefoot on the beach or in the grass.

Once you feel grounded and solid, you can look at the stressful situation and your emotions about it without feeling so overwhelmed and chaotic. You may realize that there are neutral or comforting things in the world that you can focus on to deal with your stress-related emotions. Mental imagery or using your senses to calm down can create a sense of solidness and relaxation in your brain and body. Grounding exercises signal your amygdala that you're safe in the present moment, allowing it to put the brakes on your "fight, flight, or freeze" response. Your sympathetic nervous system begins to deactivate, or your freeze begins to melt. Your breath lengthens, and your heart rate slows as your parasympathetic nervous system takes you back into a relaxed state.

Allowing and Accepting Stressful Emotions

Grounding strategies help you regain a sense of safety and normalcy when you feel overwhelmed by stress. They focus not on the emotion itself but on your senses, your imagination, or your logical mind. Both grounding and mindfulness are what researcher James Gross calls "attention allocation strategies" (Gross and Thompson 2007). When you're feeling a strong emotion, these strategies can keep you from getting caught up in it by deliberately changing the focus of your attention.

The strategies we'll discuss next take a slightly different approach to emotion. They help you let the emotion in, softening it and slowing it down so that the rest of your brain—particularly your prefrontal cortex—has time to get on board. Remember that the amygdala's position in the midbrain means that it notices stressors and sends your body into "fight, flight, or freeze" mode before your prefrontal cortex has a chance to process the information. When you slow things down, you make it less likely that stress-related fear or anger will send you into a tailspin of impulsive action or flood your mind and body with panic.

Allowing and accepting stressful emotions combines mindful awareness with a sense of exploration, curiosity, and self-compassion. Allowing emotions in involves becoming aware of any resistance you have to those emotions and gradually letting go of it. Accepting emotions means not trying to push them away or change them. It means letting them be there while you focus on noticing and describing them, rather than reacting automatically. Another word for acceptance is "willingness." To accept emotions means to be willing to experience them, even if they're uncomfortable or unwanted. Are you willing to accept the present moment and all that comes with it? As world-renowned spiritual teacher Eckhart Tolle said: "Accept—then act. Whatever the present moment contains, accept is as if you had chosen it. Always work with it, not against it. Make it your friend and ally, not your enemy. This will miraculously transform your whole life" (2004, 28).

"But why accept negative emotions such as fear and anger?" you may ask. Why be uncomfortable? Why would you want to let in emotions that lead you to behave impulsively and then face negative consequences? When you get stressed, your amygdala creates a surge of negative emotions that can make you do things you later regret, such as yelling at your boss or pressing "send" on an e-mail or text message written in a fit of rage. What if you can't stop the emotion once you let it in, and you end up collapsing in panic and distress?

The answer to these questions is simple: the emotions are there anyway. Stressful circumstances cause your amygdala to initiate a chemical cascade even before the rest of your brain knows what's going on. Brain researchers have found that there are more neural connections leading from emotional to thinking areas of the brain than the other way around. Emotions are primary, and thoughts are secondary. Emotions are wired into your brain by evolution, and you can't easily change these hardwired processes.

Second, allowing emotions in helps you learn that they're changing aspects of experience rather than fixed entities. Rather than lasting forever, emotions grow, reach a peak, and then gradually subside. Being willing to experience stressful emotions helps you get used to them, know their course, and become familiar with them. This allows your brain to see them as less dangerous or scary and more manageable and temporary. You begin to drop your aversion to them, and this makes it less likely they can lead you into a downward spiral of panic and fearful or angry reactivity.

A third reason for accepting emotions is that you can learn to separate the emotion from your negative judgments about it. The emotions involved in "fight, flight, or freeze" mode don't necessarily cause panic, but your judgments about them may. When you feel the amygdala's surge of adrenaline, you may respond with a barrage of negative judgments and aversion. If you think: *Oh my God! I can't stand this feeling!* or *I can't calm myself down. I'm going to go crazy* or *I'm so overwhelmed, I can't think straight. I just feel completely helpless!* these judgments make the feelings harder to bear.

Another reason that you need to allow and accept emotions is that emotional suppression generally doesn't work well under conditions of high stress. Trying to push away or shove down your stress-related emotions when you're very stressed actually interferes with attempts to manage stress, because suppressing your emotions can make you feel worse and increase the intensity of your stress response.

In a classic study, researchers asked one group of participants to try not to feel upset while talking about a negative event in their lives. A second group just talked about the event without suppressing their emotions (control group). The researchers then added in a stressor by asking subjects to remember a nine-digit number while speaking about the event. Under these conditions of psychological stress, emotional suppression actually increased the amount of negative emotion that participants felt about the negative event they described. It seems that trying to suppress emotions when dealing with a complex problem or difficult situation may overtax your brain's resources and cause a "rebound" effect (Wegner, Erber, and Zanakos 1993).

In another study, Case Western Reserve University psychology professor Roy Baumeister and his colleagues (1998) found that asking subjects to deliberately suppress their emotions while watching an emotional movie led them to later perform poorly on a task requiring self-control. It also led to more passive behavior. The researchers proposed that self-control gets depleted with overuse. Suppressing naturally occurring emotions requires mental effort that takes away energy and willpower that could be used to cope with the stressful situation. Chronically suppressing emotions can also take a toll on your relationships, because it makes you feel inauthentic and fake and makes other people less comfortable with you.

Many addictive behaviors, such as drinking, smoking, taking drugs, overeating, and overindulging in shopping or sex are, at their root, attempts to avoid feeling the uncomfortable emotions associated with stress. For example, people with bulimia nervosa (who binge and purge) are less aware of their emotions than people who don't have an eating disorder. Avoiding your emotions can interfere with recovery from substance abuse. If you can learn to tolerate fear, sadness, and anger, then you won't have to try to numb yourself when those emotions appear. This increases the amount of choice you have over how you're going to react and makes it more likely that you'll make a healthy choice.

In a stressful situation, mindfully accepting uncomfortable emotions helps you stay calm and present, lessening your desire to run away or zone out. It helps you feel more authentic and grounded—able to see a full picture of positive and negative emotions. This allows you to devote your full energy to goals related to dealing with the situation. If, on the other hand, you refuse to accept uncomfortable emotions, you may become passive and avoidant, meaning you may be unwilling to take reasonable risks, tolerate discomfort, or engage in certain activities if there is a chance you will feel those uncomfortable feelings. Or you may make less effective decisions because you aren't taking your emotions into account. Letting both thoughts and emotions guide you can help you cope more effectively with stressors such as unemployment, loneliness, or leaving a troubled relationship.

The Functional Side of Emotions

Evolutionary theorists believe that every emotion had a functional aspect for our ancestors, and that's why our brains are wired to experience them. Fear alerts you to a threat and gives you the energy and impetus to get away. Anger helps you protect your physical and psychological boundaries and defend yourself. Shame and regret motivate you to make different choices or to avoid repeating negative patterns. Sadness helps you conserve energy so that you can grieve. When you're under stress, you'll likely experience most, if not all, of these emotions, and it can be helpful to see them as your brain's (sometimes misguided) attempts to keep you safe, rather than as threats which need to be eliminated. For our ancestors, those who reacted more quickly to the tiger behind the bush by fighting or fleeing were more likely to live to tell the tale and have their offspring survive. Thus, an active amygdala gave them an evolutionary advantage in a world where the major sources of stress were wild animals and famine. Over time, "fight, flight, or freeze" mode got hardwired into our brains as an automatic response to stressful circumstances.

If our amygdala is there to protect us, why can't we just listen to its message of alarm and follow its impulse to action? Although this strategy may work in extreme situations—such as when you're being followed down a dark alley at night or when you encounter a rattlesnake—in other situations, blindly obeying your amygdala may actually veer you off course from your long-term goals. The problem is that your amygdala has an "on" and "off" switch rather than a graduated dial. It reacts in an "all or nothing" way. But the stresses of the modern world are complex. Running away, fighting, or freezing doesn't serve you well when you're facing a stressor such as loneliness, unemployment, unpaid bills, or difficult negotiations. But if you can allow in the emotions without acting impulsively or pushing them away, they can alert you to a threat or important factor you need to pay attention to.

PRACTICE: Allowing In Your Emotions

Sit down in a quiet place, and let your breath settle. Take a few breaths, following your breath through your body as you breathe in and breathe out. Now think about a stressful situation that you're currently facing. Find an image in your mind's eye that represents the worst or most important aspect of the situation—for example, visualize a pile of unpaid bills or the face of an irate boss. Focus on the image until it's really clear. Now notice how the image makes you feel in your body.

Now check in with your body and notice any areas of discomfort, tightness, or tingling. You may notice these sensations in your head, neck, shoulders, chest, solar plexus, belly, feet, or other parts of your body. Notice any feelings of anxiety, panic, or being "speeded up" (such as your heart racing or your breathing getting shallower). These are signs that your amygdala has sent your sympathetic nervous system into "fight, flight, or freeze" mode. Now try to name these sensations—for example, say silently (or aloud) "My chest is tight" or "I feel butterflies in my stomach."

Now try to attach an emotion word to these body sensations. Are you feeling fear, anger, sadness, guilt, shame, or a mixture of these? Say silently (or aloud) "I'm feeling fear" or "I'm angry" (for example). At the same time, notice if you have any aversion or resistance to this emotion. Notice any negative labels or judgments you attach to the emotion, such as "I can't stand feeling this way" or "Why can't I just get over it?" After acknowledging that these judgments are there, try to hold them a bit more lightly and refocus your attention on your bodily sensations. Notice the difference between the emotion itself and your resistance to it. Say to yourself, *It's okay to let myself feel this emotion.*

Focus again on the emotion in your body and notice whether the emotion in your body has changed or stayed the same. Is there any difference in intensity since the beginning of this practice? Stay with the emotion for a few more moments and then bring your attention slowly back to the room. Do you see the stressful situation any differently?

Allowing in emotions is a mindfulness practice, in that you're deliberately focusing your attention on your emotions with an attitude of openness and curiosity. You're also noticing the difference between the emotion itself and your aversion or judgments about it and trying to hold your judgments more lightly. If you practice several times a week, you'll become more familiar and comfortable with your day-to-day and stress-related emotions and the bodily sensations that accompany them. A mindful attitude will help slow you down and will create a sense of calm, so that you're less likely to act impulsively or get into a mindspin or state of panic.

Allowing emotions in will help you notice, understand, and describe how you feel about your stressful situation. If you ever fear that an emotion will go on forever or make you crazy, the next practice will help you learn that emotions are temporary: any emotion you experience will reach a peak and then recede.

PRACTICE: Surfing the Wave of Your Emotions

In the book *Wherever You Go, There You Are: Mindfulness Meditation in Everyday Life* (1994), mindfulness pioneer Jon Kabat-Zinn said that mindfulness is like surfing the waves of your emotions. You can't stop the waves from coming, but you can learn to surf so that you don't get knocked down by them.

1. Sit comfortably on a chair, a couch, or the floor, and maintain an upright yet relaxed pose. Begin to bring your attention to your breath, watching it go in and out. Notice the pause between the breaths. Do this for a few breaths.

2. Begin thinking about your stressful situation. Try to get a clear image that represents the worst or most important aspect of your stressor.

3. Notice what you feel in your body and where you feel it, and give the emotion a name, such as "anger" or "sadness." You may feel more than one feeling, and that's fine.

4. Rate the intensity of your feeling, from neutral (0) to extremely intense (10). After you have a number in mind, keep watching the feeling in your body while continuing to breathe. Just notice the feeling and try to adopt an open, accepting, curious attitude toward it. If you notice any tightness or tension, send some breath into that area of your body. Notice any judgments you have about the feeling, and try to hold them less tightly or picture them floating away.

5. Keep watching the feeling, noticing any change in intensity over time. Do this for fifteen to twenty minutes, noting the intensity every five minutes or so.

Did the feeling get more intense and rise to a crescendo, then gradually fade away?

Once you have the "emotion surfing" technique down, you can begin to use it when you feel a difficult emotion arising or when you have to do something that makes you feel uncomfortable. Whenever you have to confront somebody, fill out a tax return, give a speech, go on a first date, write an exam, or interview for a job, notice what you feel in your body and name the emotion. Putting emotions into words also makes the right hemisphere of your brain (which is more spatial and holistic) work together with the left hemisphere (which is more linguistic and detail-oriented). Thus you can bring in your whole brain and create a more balanced reaction to the stressor.

Allowing emotions in without judging or changing them can make you more comfortable with your emotions, but you can also work more directly on containing, softening, and soothing emotions. In the next section, you'll learn a few different ways to do this.

Containing, Softening, and Soothing Your Emotions

Having a stress-proof brain means that you can experience emotions about your stressful situation in a balanced way, without letting "fight, flight, or freeze" mode take over and knock you off balance or cause you to act unwisely. Knowing how to soften and soothe your stress-related emotions so that you can hear their message more calmly and clearly can be very advantageous. You also probably want to know how to keep stress-related emotions contained so that they don't take over your mind and body. In the following practices, you'll use mental imagery to help you calm your amygdala's "fight, flight, or freeze" response and the fearful or angry emotions it creates.

PRACTICE: Softening Emotions in Your Body

Sit down in a quiet place, and let your breath settle. Take a few breaths, following your breath as you breathe in and out. Now think about your stressful situation. Find an image in your mind's eye that represents the worst or most important aspect of the situation—for example, visualize a pile of unpaid bills or the face of an irate boss. Focus on the image until it's really clear.

Now notice how the image makes you feel in your body. Try to locate the exact sensation in your body, and just notice it. Try to describe it in words: "a lump in my throat," "heat in my head," and so on. What emotion is it signaling? Consider that emotion. What is it like? What color would it be, if it had one? Is it large in size, medium, or small? Is it heavy or light? And what shape is it? Does it have edges? Are those edges smooth or jagged? And how does it feel—warm or cold? Does it feel rough or smooth? Finally, is the emotion stationary or is it moving? If it's moving, does it move quickly or slowly?

Once you've answered these questions, visualize the emotion in your body in terms of these qualities. You might imagine a heavy gray blob, a green puddle of goo, a broken heart, or streaks of light. In this way, you're using mental imagery and your intuitive senses to give form and sensory qualities to the emotion so that you can work with it.

Now try to find a way to soften this emotion. If the edges are jagged, can you smooth them out a bit? If the emotion is heavy, can you make it a bit lighter? If it's large, can you shrink it a bit? If it's dense, can you make it a bit more permeable? You might also imagine softening the shape at the edges or wrapping it up in a soft, cloud-like material. You might ask it what it needs and see whether you get an answer. Continue to look for ways to soften the emotion, and keep noticing how the emotion changes. When it won't soften any more, stop and slowly come back to the room. You may find that the emotion is less dense in your body, less intense, and less threatening than when you began.

In the next practice, you'll learn another way of soothing an emotion by using nature imagery to picture it as a moving, flowing object. This creates a bit of distance from the emotion, which makes you realize that the emotion is not *you*. The images I've chosen are similar to those used in many mindfulness trainings.

PRACTICE: Using Nature Imagery to Externalize the Emotion

This practice involves using your imagination to get to know your stress-related emotions with an attitude of mindfulness and open curiosity. Choose the images you like the best, or try out all of them.

A pond. Imagine that your mind is a pond in the middle of the forest. On the surface, the water is brown, muddy, and murky, with twigs, debris, and fallen leaves. Imagine that your emotions about the stressful situation are the objects on the surface that churn up the water and make it cloudy. Watch them slowly settle down until the water is cool, calm, and clear and you can see the bottom of the pond. When you let your feelings of stress settle, you can see the situation with greater clarity and peace of mind! (The pond or lake image in mindfulness meditation was used in "The Lake Meditation" in Jon Kabat-Zinn's 1994 book *Wherever You Go, There You Are: Mindfulness Meditation in Everyday Life*).

An ocean. Imagine that your mind is a cool, blue ocean, and your stressful emotions are waves. Imagine the waves rising and cresting, then breaking with a crash of white foam, and then slowly getting weaker and calmer. Watch the waves as they rise and fall.

The sky. Imagine that your mind is the sky and your emotions are clouds floating by. Give the clouds a different character, depending on the type of emotion and its intensity. There might be ominous, gray storm clouds for anger and little white puffy ones for happy feelings. Notice which emotions draw you in and which ones you want to push away. Even if you feel attached to them, practice letting go and just letting them float on by to make room for the next one.

A storm. Imagine that your emotions are rain and wind, washing over you. Notice how the storm gets more intense, with heavy drops and fierce winds, how it reaches a peak, and then how it gradually calms down until you're left with a few tiny, light raindrops. You can imagine a rainbow at the end if you like.

A fire. Imagine that your emotions are a fire, and you're watching it from a safe distance. Notice the flames get fiercer and crackle loudly before gradually dying down until you're left with smoking embers.

Expressing Your Emotions

Another way to deal with your emotions about your stressful situation is to find a safe way to express them. You can express them by drawing, writing in a journal, or confiding in a trusted friend or family member. University of Texas psychology professor James Pennebaker is a pioneer in the field of emotional expression. He created a brief self-help intervention (Pennebaker and Chung 2011) that involves writing down your deepest thoughts and emotions about an unresolved or ongoing stressful event. He also asks subjects to "write a narrative with a beginning, middle, and end" and to link the facts of the event with the corresponding thoughts and emotions. Subjects write for twenty to thirty minutes on each of three or four days.

This writing intervention has been tested in hundreds of studies looking at people undergoing all kinds of stressors (Frattaroli 2006), and it has helped people stay healthy, feel better, and take positive action. There have, however, been some studies that found no beneficial effects and some studies in which writing helped some people more than others. In one study, recently laid-off engineers and managers who wrote expressively about their job loss were more likely to find employment in the next few months than those who didn't do this type of writing (Spera, Buhrfeind, and Pennebaker 1994). The authors of the study suggested that negative emotions and anger about the job loss might "leak out" and interfere with positive motivation to get a new job and performance at the interview. Writing may have helped resolve these emotions.

In another study, which I conducted with my colleague, Columbia University health and behavioral studies professor Stephen J. Lepore (Lepore and Greenberg 2002), college students who wrote down their thoughts and emotions about a recent relationship breakup were more likely to get back together with their ex partner than the group that was asked to write about non-emotional events (such as attitudes toward college dating). Although the number of ex-partners getting back together was small overall, expressive writing may have helped those who wanted to reunite be more proactive about it. Also, those who wrote expressively about the breakup had less tension and fatigue and fewer respiratory symptoms (such as coughing and sneezing) in subsequent weeks. Perhaps writing helped them realize that the breakup was inevitable or for the best, so they felt less stressed.

Expressive writing has helped students adjust to college and face the stress of final exams. Four months after participating in an expressive writing intervention in which they wrote about stressful events, patients with asthma had improved lung function, and patients with rheumatoid arthritis received better health ratings from physicians (Smyth et al. 1999). Similarly, after writing about the stress of cancer, cancer patients reported fewer physical symptoms and made fewer physician visits for cancer-related problems (Stanton et al. 2002).

Why does expressive writing help you stay healthy when faced with many different kinds of stressors? Writing may help you overcome your avoidance and procrastination and face what you're feeling, as well as helping you better understand what you want and need from the stressful situation. This can give you more clarity and encourage you to be proactive in creating and pursuing goals related to the stressor. Creating a narrative that integrates the facts of the stressful situation with thoughts and emotions may have a grounding effect, which helps your amygdala calm down so that you can act more effectively. Such a narrative may give you new insight and perspective that can help you feel less distressed about the situation. Writing in twenty-to-thirty-minute increments gives you a time-limited way to focus on and externalize your emotions about the stressor. Just as writing a "to do" list helps you tackle one task at a time, writing about your stressor helps you face your emotions about the situation in small "doses," rather than all at once. Ready to give it a try?

PRACTICE: Expressing Your Thoughts and Emotions in Writing

Get a pen and paper ready, or buy an attractive journal to write in. Sit down in a quiet place where you won't be disturbed. Switch off your cell phone and other electronic devices.

Then, for the next twenty to thirty minutes, write about the stressful event you're facing. Be sure to include the facts of the event, together with your thoughts and emotions about it. Try to write a narrative with a clear beginning, middle, and end. Don't worry about spelling, handwriting, or grammar. The important thing is that you write about your deepest thoughts and emotions. (If you find the writing too distressing, it's okay to take a break or stop.) Try to do the same thing the next day and the following day, or make your journal a regular part of your life.

If you have experienced a serious trauma, such as sexual abuse, and have very intense feelings about it or are highly avoidant of facing it, you may want to consult a trained mental health professional, rather than relying solely on self-help methods such as expressive writing.

Final Thoughts

In this chapter, you learned that in a stressful situation it's unhelpful to suppress your emotions, because they can rebound. Emotional suppression also requires willpower and energy that you could better use to manage your stressors.

Emotions contain valuable information about your reactions to a situation. They also can help you take action to protect yourself, conserve your energy, or learn from experience. If you're willing to accept your emotions—even if they make you uncomfortable—they'll rise, reach a peak, and then gradually subside. Thinking of your emotions as a wave or rainstorm can be helpful.

Expressing your emotions in a diary or journal will help you tie them to the events that created them and your thoughts about the situation. This may help you feel calmer. It may also lead to new insights or coping strategies that can help you better manage your stressors.

CHAPTER 5

Gaining Control over Your Stress

When you're faced with a lengthy stressor or a series of stressful problems, you may feel as if you're losing control over your life: you try really hard to cope, but, despite your best efforts, nothing seems to change. Not having control over important events in your life can exacerbate feelings of stress and cause depression. Problems that you can't do anything about are more likely to trigger "fight, flight, or freeze" mode than problems that seem controllable. Luckily, there are ways to perceive some control over your stressor, even in the most trying of circumstances. In this chapter, you'll learn how to feel more in control of your life stressors. Even if you can't control all of your stressors, you'll learn to focus on the parts you can control. You'll use your prefrontal cortex to reevaluate the stressful circumstances or your coping abilities and then feed the information back to your amygdala to calm it down.

Why Control Is Important

Humans have a strong preference for controllable conditions. For our ancestors, unpredictability, uncertainty, and lack of control were dangerous. They needed to know when predators were likely to be asleep or away so that they could plan their trips to get food and water in safety. They needed to know the best times to plant and harvest their crops so that they could store enough food and supplies to last the winter. If things were out of place or not as expected, it could mean grave danger. Over thousands of years, the need to feel in control became wired into our human brains. Our amygdalae are designed to view lack of control and unpredictability as threats to survival and to react by triggering the stress response. Unfortunately, change and uncertainty are facts of life in the modern world. Terrorists, economic collapse, earthquakes, and murders flash across our TV screens, constantly sending our amygdalae into high alert.

Humans aren't the only creatures who get more stressed if they don't have control. As you'll learn in this chapter, research with rodents, dogs, monkeys, and other animals clearly demonstrates that uncontrollable stress is more toxic to the brain, body, and behavior of many species than controllable stress. In the classic "learned helplessness" study (Seligman and Maier 1967), dogs were exposed either to electric shocks they could terminate by pushing a lever (controllable shock condition) or to electric shocks that began and ended independently of the dogs' behavior (uncontrollable shock condition). Although both groups received the same overall amount of shock, dogs that were exposed to uncontrollable shock acted more distressed. Even more troubling, when the dogs were later put into a shuttle box in which they could escape shock by jumping over a barrier, only those previously exposed to controllable shock successfully learned the escape response. Dogs who had been previously exposed to uncontrollable shock did not learn to escape the shock. The researchers theorized that the dogs in the uncontrollable shock condition had previously learned that their behaviors could not prevent the aversive consequences, so they gave up trying. Thus, they never learned that conditions had changed and that escape was now within reach. Professor Seligman believed that these problems in learning and motivation were similar to those found in people with depression. He proposed that depression is a form of "learned helplessness" caused by uncontrollable stress in early life.

Rodent studies also suggest strongly that uncontrollable stress both is more stressful and has more toxic aftereffects than controllable stress: rodents that were exposed to uncontrollable shock showed greater deficits in learning and more stress-related changes in brain neurotransmitters than rodents that had an opportunity to terminate the shock by pushing a lever and no-shock controls (Altenor, Kay, and Richter 1977; Weiss, Stone, and Harrell 1970; Weiss et al. 1975). In addition, rodents that were shocked at random intervals were more stressed and exhibited more toxic effects than those shocked at regular, predictable intervals (Mineka and Kihlstrom 1978). Knowing when the shock was coming allowed them a period of relative safety to recover between shocks.

Uncontrollable stress seems to interfere with our natural motivation to seek out new and interesting experiences. Baby monkeys reared in environments where they can control access to food, water, and treats later show less fear and more exploratory behavior when placed in an unfamiliar situation than monkeys reared in uncontrollable environments (Mineka, Gunnar, and Champoux 1986). In humans, as you learned earlier, uncontrollable stress in childhood can damage the prefrontal cortex's ability to modulate the amygdala's stress response. Humans who were exposed to chronic, uncontrollable stress as children may be more passive and less motivated to try out new ways of thinking and behaving that could help them adapt to stressful circumstances.

One area where you may experience uncontrollable stress is at work. Most workers can't control their work demands, their salary, how the boss treats them, the assignments they receive, or when they have to work. The Whitehall Studies in Great Britain (mentioned in chapter 2; Marmot et al. 1991) examined the relationship between job grade, perceived control, and long-term health in more than ten thousand British civil servants (government employees). Those in the higher job grades (such as managers and executives) had a much lower rate of overall mortality (chance of dying) and heart disease than those in lower grades. They also perceived much more control over their work, and the more control they felt, the better their health. In general, the most stressful jobs are those in which you have high levels of responsibility but low levels of control. It's not the executive in the back office but the administrative assistant at the front desk who generally is more stressed.

If you're dealing with uncontrollable stress, you should feel happy that you bought this book. Research shows that if you can find some way to perceive control over your stressful circumstances, you'll be less likely to be negatively affected by them and more likely to cope effectively (Rodin 1986; Thompson et al. 1993). How you view your stressor is just as important as your actual circumstances when it comes to long-term effects on your health and happiness!

Trying to find perceived control may, at first, seem antithetical to mindfulness. In the previous chapter, you learned about mindfully facing and accepting your emotions, rather than deliberately trying to change them. But mindfulness can coexist with strengthening your sense of control. The idea is that you mindfully accept what's happening in the present but also face the stressor actively and take thoughtful action to address the stressor. You also try to distinguish between the things you can influence and those you can't, using mindfulness to accept what you can't change. Mindfulness is not the same as passive acceptance. Rather, it involves working actively to let go of aversion and judgments that make you feel more helpless and out of control.

How You View Your Stress Matters

In addition to stressful events themselves, your attitude toward your stress can affect your mood and health. If you have to give a presentation and you feel your heart racing and butterflies in your stomach, you may start feeling really stressed and focus on everything that might go wrong. But if you interpret these same feelings as signs of excitement, you'll feel less stressed and more focused on your passion for the topic or sharing your expert knowledge.

The Perceived Stress Scale (PSS) developed by Dr. Sheldon Cohen and colleagues at Carnegie Mellon University (Cohen, Kamarck, and Mermelstein 1983) measures the degree to which you feel out of control and overwhelmed by the circumstances of your life. It asks questions such as "In the last month, how often have you felt that you could not cope with all the things that you had to do?" and "In the past month, how often have you felt nervous and stressed?" High levels of perceived stress have been shown to predict heart disease, depression, anxiety, and many other negative health outcomes associated with chronic stress, such as lowered immunity. On the other hand, finding ways to feel less stressed, even in relatively uncontrollable circumstances, can protect your brain and body.

Why does your attitude toward stress make such a difference? If you feel as if you're facing the end of the world, you create chronic worry that interferes with your parasympathetic nervous system's ability to switch off "fight, flight, or freeze" mode when the stressor isn't present. Your thoughts and feelings about the stressor will intrude on other aspects of your life. Remember that our brains and bodies were designed to alternate periods of feeling activated with a chance to rest and replenish our energy. So when your sick toddler is finally taking a nap, your angry partner has finally calmed down, finals are over, your taxes are paid, or you've survived the traffic on the expressway and are safely home at night, you need to let your brain know that you're entering a period of safety and no longer need to fight, freeze, or flee. Your brain needs to switch off the stress response so that you won't have as much spillover into the parts of your life that aren't supposed to be stressful!

If you had a lot of uncontrollable stress in childhood, your perceptions of stress are likely being fed by beliefs and feelings related to these past events. The way our brains learn what to fear plays a big part in this process. Our brains create strong and salient memories of what's unsafe, and they keep bringing those memories up in situations that are even slightly similar. For example, if you were abandoned as a child, you may fear abandonment by your partner. As a result, you may either avoid romantic relationships altogether or, more likely, feel stressed and triggered every time you fight with your partner or every time your partner seems to be distancing himself or herself from you.

Once your brain has learned that a certain kind of situation (such as being in a relationship) is dangerous, it's very hard for it to unlearn that information and regard that kind of situation as safe. Avoidance blocks opportunities for new learning, as you saw in the learned help-lessness paradigm. It's also due to the way your amygdala operates. Your amygdala has only an "on and off" switch, not a dial with different levels. So your amygdala will sound the alarm when you get into any type of situation that's similar to the one that previously stressed you. Your amygdala tends to overgeneralize—it's not good at seeing differences. For example, if you failed your math exam, your amygdala might still create strong stress signals when you write your history essay, even though you're an A student in history. That's why you can't just rely on your amygdala—you have to take a mindful break and slow down so that your prefrontal cortex can get on board and send feedback to switch off "fight, flight, or freeze" mode when you're overreacting.

Getting stressed about your stress will only make it worse. Stress is a fact of life that has to be managed, not eliminated. As you learned in chapter 1, acute stress can energize you to perform at your best and even help you grow new brain neurons! In one study (Crum, Salovey, and Achor 2013), people who perceived their stress as damaging to their health actually had more health problems than people who perceived the same level of stress less negatively. The secret is to find a way to see your stressful situation as at least partially under your control and to feel more confident in your skills and coping abilities.

Building Stress Resilience

Research shows that overcoming some level of stress and adversity can make us more resilient in the future. Researchers at the University of California (Seery, Holman, and Silver 2010) followed a national sample of participants for several years. They found the usual negative effects of very high stress exposure, as well as something surprising: people who had experienced some adversity (such as the death of a loved one) reported being less stressed by recent life events and had fewer mental health problems than those who had previously experienced no adversity. Stress that you can control or master seems to have an "inoculation" effect. What doesn't kill you can make you stronger. You may be more likely to have confidence in your coping abilities—to see yourself as someone who can overcome life's difficulties.

One of the first researchers to investigate resilience was University of California child psychologist Emmy Werner (Werner and Smith 2001). She and her colleagues studied a group of children who had experienced poverty, victimization, and neglect, and they tracked these children to age forty. Two-thirds of the children didn't fare well in life. But the rest grew into happy, successful, healthy, and optimistic adults. The researchers noticed that the children who fared well had some "protective factors" in common. Besides a good temperament, they had been able to find at least one adult outside the family who acted as a caring and positive role model. They also had at least one skill (such as skill at sports, music, or academics) that gave them a sense of pride and achievement and led peers and teachers to view them positively.

If there's an area of your life in which you can experience a sense of control and feel good about your achievements, then stress in other areas won't drag you down as much. Try to find a hobby, volunteer activity, or sport that gives you a sense of accomplishment. Many top executives are also runners, and they credit running with helping them get through difficult times. If household errands and responsibilities cause you to feel stressed, then volunteering at your kids' school, coaching their sports team, or doing service in your community can provide a sense of control and accomplishment that buffers you against that stress. Baking, scrapbooking, painting, hiking, working out, or writing a blog can also create a sense of self-worth and positive achievement.

Applying Perceived Control to Reduce Your Stress

As mentioned, your amygdala isn't good at differentiating between similar situations. It just tells you there's a situation that you'd better pay attention to and initiates "fight, flight, or freeze" mode. Your prefrontal cortex, on the other hand, can take a more sophisticated view of the situation and let your amygdala know "We've got this. You can relax." Research shows that perceiving control over at least some part of your life circumstances can help make you less physically and psychologically reactive to stress (Neupert, Almeida, and Charles 2007; Wallston et al. 1987).

Our perceived level of control seems to go down as we age, perhaps because we're more likely to experience serious illness, declining abilities, or the death of a loved one. Elderly nursing home residents, for example, experience strong feelings of stress and very little actual control over their lives. Elderly people who enter nursing homes often become less active and more depressed and apathetic. A classic study (Langer and Rodin 1976; Rodin and Langer 1977) beautifully illustrates the power of increasing perceived control over life circumstances. In this study of elderly nursing-home residents, participants in one group were given an intervention designed to increase perceived control over their lives: they were told that they had control over and should take personal responsibility for their participation in activities, socializing, and daily routine. They were also each given a plant and instructed to water it. Participants in the other group received a "low control" intervention: they were told that the nursing-home staff would look after them. They were given a plant as well, but they were told that it would be watered by the nursing-home staff.

The results were striking! Over the next eighteen months, participants in the high-control group were more active, had better health, demonstrated less deterioration in mood and sociability, and were less likely to die than those in the low-control group. Perceiving more control apparently led the residents to make more effort and participate more in activities. They were therefore more likely to find natural rewards, such as friendships and new knowledge, which may have created a positive cycle of engaging and feeling good. I love this study, because I still have a mental picture of my elderly mother in her small but sunny apartment filled to the brim with plants that she cared for herself (without knowing about this study). Despite facing many stressful situations in her life, she lived to be ninety-one!

There are a couple of different ways to perceive control over your stressful circumstances. You may believe that you can do something to beneficially affect the outcome of your stress. If you're in a troubled stage of your relationship but believe that you (and your partner) can restore intimacy, you'll feel less stressed. If you're facing a difficult test and believe that studying hard will lead to success, your stress level will go down. Unemployed people who continue to believe that they'll find a job or other opportunity and that the unemployment is only temporary have better mental health than those who don't have confidence they'll find a job.

Researchers have studied the effects of perceived control in medical populations and found that perceiving control over your symptoms or the outcome of your illness makes you more resilient. Studies of patients coping with the stress of arthritis, chronic pain, or fibromyalgia report more depression and disability if they feel helpless to control their symptoms or illness (Hommel et al. 2001; Palomino et al. 2007; Casey et al. 2008). This effect occurs over and above any differences in severity of symptoms or medical treatments. Stress can provoke symptom flare-ups in these types of illnesses, and feeling help-less increases your stress levels. On the other hand, feeling in control of your disease or symptoms makes you less stressed and more likely to stay active and functional. One way to feel in control is to see yourself as a person who can do (or learn to do) what the situation calls for.

Finding the Confidence to Manage Your Stress

Research (for example, Curtis, Groarke, and Sullivan 2014) shows that if you feel confident you can manage your stress, you'll feel less stressed. Having a role model who faced the same difficulties and coped suc-cessfully is one way to boost your confidence. For example, if you want to get sober, attending Alcoholics Anonymous meetings is likely to improve your confidence that you can remain sober over the long haul, because the older members act as positive role models for the newcom-ers by sharing their stories of sobriety or of getting back on track after a relapse. Do you have a role model or know somebody who has mas-tered a similar stressor? Reaching out to that person and asking for advice can improve your confidence and coping skills.

Think about your stressful circumstances and your level of confi-dence that you can do something constructive to cope, meet your goals, or avoid a negative outcome. Some questions to ask yourself are:

- *What helped me survive other difficult circumstances in my life?*

- *Have I faced this type of situation before?*

- *What skills or personal qualities do I possess that might help me manage the situation?*

- *What external resources or support can I rely on to help me deal with the stressor?*

A client whom I'll call Susan (actually a composite and not a real client) was in the throes of a divorce and felt very stressed at the prospect of marital breakup, financial struggle, and single parenthood. I led her step by step through these questions, and she remembered how she had survived a childhood with an alcoholic mother. She had successfully coped with a previous relationship breakup by joining a gym, moving from the suburbs to the city (where she would meet more potential partners), and reminding herself of her self-worth. She thought about how thrifty she had been during college and realized that she could be happy with fewer material things. Susan also realized that she was a good parent and well able to take care of her son when her ex-husband traveled for work. Her sister and friends could provide emotional support and babysitting help. And she was, above all, a survivor! By consciously bringing to mind past experiences of stress mastery and current resources she could rely on, Susan was able to increase her self-confidence and feel more control over her life. This led her to feel less stressed and more optimistic.

PRACTICE: Finding Confidence to Manage Your Stressor

Answer the following questions in a journal or on a separate piece of paper.

1. What's the stressful situation you're facing?

2. On a scale of 0 (no confidence) to 10 (complete confidence), rate your level of confidence in your ability to manage the situation.

3. Explain your rating. Why do you believe that you can or can't manage this situation successfully?

4. Have you faced any major stress, trauma, or adversity in your life? If so, what skills, efforts, or personal qualities helped you get through it?

5. Can you apply any of these qualities, efforts, or skills in your current situation? How?

6. Do you know of anybody who has faced a similar situation and gotten through it successfully?

7. Have you faced the same type of situation (such as a similar breakup or a similarly demanding job) in the past? If so, how did you get through it?

8. Is there anything you've learned from your previous experiences with stress that can help you in this situation? How have your knowledge and skills improved since the last time you experienced this type of event?

9. What other resources, support, or tools can you use to manage this situation? (For example, can you get help from friends or family? Can you do Internet research? Can you rely on your courage?)

Now that you've answered these questions, rate your current level of confidence in your ability to manage the situation. Is there any change since the first rating? Explain.

Although confidence to cope is beneficial, perceiving unrealistic control in low-control circumstances can be a double-edged sword. Persisting too much when it would be more productive to try a different tack can lead to frustration and burnout. Not every aspect of your situation is controllable. Yet feeling completely out of control creates more stress hormones and makes you more likely to give up. Therefore it's best to make realistic judgments about what you can and can't control. In the next section, you'll learn to be strategic in the way you perceive control.

Deciding Which Parts of the Stressor You Can Control

Now that you know how important it is to feel a sense of control over your stressor, how do you go about doing this? Sometimes it's easy. If you're running a marathon, you can decide which race you want to run in, set a training schedule, and then just do it. On the other hand, if you're facing a contentious divorce, a cancer diagnosis, a long period of unemployment, infertility, or the loss of a loved one, or if you have an alcoholic or drug-addicted family member, you have less actual control over the final outcome. If you believe you have control of the whole process and you really don't, you might end up having unrealistic goals or engaging in wishful thinking and getting very frustrated when things don't turn out as you wanted. This can lead you to wear yourself out or blame yourself for things that weren't your doing.

How do you avoid the pitfalls of perceiving unrealistic control while taking advantage of the positive, stress-reducing aspects of perceiving realistic control? One way is to perceive control over the process or the outcome of your efforts. For example, if you're organizing a charity or school event, you can remind yourself that you're an organized person, that you've given yourself enough time, and that you've gotten enough help, so you know the event will be successful even if there are a few minor glitches. This feeling can keep you going through the interminable phone calls, e-mails, and negotiations with vendors. When I moved from San Diego to Marin County, California, to start my clinical psychology practice, I didn't know the area or the people. Nevertheless, I felt confident in my competence, credentials, and ability to promote my practice. I also knew that building a business takes perseverance. Having realistic expectations and confidence in my abilities reduced my level of stress. In the following practice, you'll have the opportunity to define which parts of your stressor are controllable and develop a plan of action.

PRACTICE: Deciding What You Can and Can't Control

Think about the stressful situation you're facing. Consider different aspects of the situation, and list them in a journal or on a separate piece of paper. If they're mostly under your control, write them under "Things I Can Control." If they're mostly not under your control, write them under "Things I Can't Control." If you're not sure, write them under "Not Sure."

For example, if you're facing stress at work because of a demanding boss, you might create the following lists.

Things I Can Control

How many hours I work

The quality of my work

Getting the work done on time

Delegating some tasks

Asking for help if I need it

Getting enough rest and exercise so that I can focus

Preparing for the presentation

Things I Can't Control

My boss's demands and priorities

Work deadlines

My job assignments

How much staff I currently have

Whether the client is happy

Not Sure

Skills of my team. I can work to increase these if I have enough time.

Extra resources. I can ask my boss for more resources, but I don't know whether I'll get them.

Once you understand which pieces you can control and which you can't, make a plan to address the controllable aspects. Break tasks down and schedule specific times to work on them. Set a realistic timetable, and keep yourself accountable. Anticipate obstacles and distractions, and make a plan to deal with them. If you find yourself ruminating about the uncontrollable aspects, either deliberately refocus on the controllable stuff or get up and do something else.

Letting Go of What You Can't Control

Although you can feel in control of the effort you put in and how much you build your skills, you can't always control the final result. We can't control what other people feel or do, the state of the economy or politics, the weather, what the competition is like, or whether our skills or products are currently in vogue. That's why it's important to set goals and evaluate your progress in terms of your effort, rather than outcome. Don't focus on getting an A; focus on being well-prepared and knowledgeable about the topic. Don't focus on getting a job; focus on getting your applications out, networking, staying healthy and positive, and getting the skills and information you need. Don't focus on finding the perfect partner; focus on looking and feeling your best and getting out in the world where you're likely to meet potential mates.

When outcomes are uncertain, most of us spend a great deal of energy ruminating, worrying, and second-guessing ourselves. Not only is this a waste of time, but it makes us less likely to succeed. Ruminating actually brings down our mood and makes us less likely to go out and do something about the stressor. The following practice will help you keep the things you can't control mentally contained, to limit their intrusion into your life.

PRACTICE: **Putting Things You Can't Control into a Container**

Once you've defined the parts of the problem that you can't control, the next step is to deliberately move your attention away from these aspects so that you can focus on doing the best job you can with the controllable pieces of your stressor. Of course, you can't completely control your worries, but you can let your amygdala know you have the uncontrollable stuff contained. That way, your brain will be less likely to remind you of everything that might go wrong!

This practice is adapted from the Training Manual of Dr. Philip Manfield, who is one of my clinical mentors and an expert in eye movement desensitization and reprocessing (EMDR) treatment for trauma. Use it whenever you feel yourself getting caught up in worrying about outcomes that are out of your control, to free yourself to devote your time and energy to the things you *can* control.

Before you begin, if you could hold your worries and fears about the uncontrollable parts of your stressor in a container of some sort, what type of container would you choose? Examples of containers are a big oak barrel, a sturdy trunk, a metal safe, and a large vase.

1. Once you have decided on a container, bring up a mental picture of it. Be very specific about its size, shape, color, and texture. You may want to imagine labeling your container with descriptions such as "Fears About My Divorce." You can also imagine writing or drawing on the container or decorating it in whichever way you choose.

2. Imagine putting all of your worries and fears about uncontrollable outcomes of your stress into the container. Visualize yourself packing them in, or see your worries as a stream of smoke, light, sand, or water that flows into the container. Give them the form that feels right to you.

3. Once all your worries are in the container, imagine sealing it. You could use a lid, a lock, chains, plastic wrap, or all of the above. It's up to you. When your container is sealed tight, imagine storing it somewhere. You could bury it deep underground, put it in a cave, stow it in an attic, load it onto a boat, or send it into space in a rocket ship. Anywhere you want to store it is okay.

4. When your container is sealed and stored, imagine yourself walking away from it and back into your life. You can come back and open it if you need to, but for now it's safely put away.

5. Set an intention to focus your effort and energy on the parts of your stressor that you *can* control.

Even if you don't have control over the outcome of a stressful situation, you may be able to exert some control over its impact. If you have chronic pain, chronic anxiety, or an illness you can't control, set goals that relate to staying active or moving forward despite the pain, symptoms, or anxiety. Many patients make the mistake of trying to find a "cure" for a condition that's chronic and needs to be managed. You can't always control what you feel or think, but you can control what you do! Focus on living a full life even though you don't have a partner. Or focus on being the best parent or partner you can be, despite having a stressful job or spending most of your day carpooling and doing laundry. Find ways to have fun with your family and friends, even if you don't have a lot of money.

A concept related to that of control is that of meaningfulness. When your life feels full and meaningful despite your having stress or not being able to get everything done, you'll feel a greater sense of control over your life circumstances. Think about what really is most important and meaningful in your life. Is it your close relationships, achievement, making a difference in the world, helping others, being a good parent, contributing to your community, helping the environment, living by certain values, being an innovator, or living a healthy life? When you decide what's most important in life and set realistic goals in that area, your brain will register that your life is under control. Stress is a fact of life, but it doesn't have to consume you.

Finally, like the resilient kids in Werner and Smith's study or the nursing-home residents who watered their own plants, you can focus on developing a skill or interest that's separate from the stress and under your control. This can create a sense of accomplishment that counterbalances your stress.

PRACTICE: Finding Control in Other Areas of Your Life

This practice will help you identify an aspect of your life unrelated to the stressor, an area of your life in which you can grow. Think about a sport, a hobby, an activity, or a relationship that's important to you, ideally something you can focus on for twenty minutes to an hour or two at a time. Think about why you value this activity and how doing it will give you a sense of pride, control, and accomplishment. It could be volunteer work, art, writing, baking or cooking, scrapbooking, running, hiking, joining a yoga class, meditating, spending time with your partner (or parent or child), or anything else that's personally important to you.

Now decide how much time you want to dedicate to this activity, or figure out what you want to achieve in the next week, the next month, and so on. For example, I set myself the goal of getting fitter by climbing the hills in my neighborhood for thirty minutes a day, three times a week, for one month. Once I had achieved this, I set a goal for the next month to do this four times a week. A client of mine set a goal of trying out a new recipe every Sunday, while another signed up for a 5K Fun Run and began training for it. A friend of mine set a goal of clearing a closet or drawer of clutter every week. Write down your goal, and check your progress toward it at least once a week. Pick something you can realistically do. If you need to adjust your goal as you go along, that's fine. Each day, remind yourself that despite your stressful circumstances, you're making clear progress in a personally important life area. Allow yourself to feel proud of what you've achieved.

Final Thoughts

In this chapter, you learned about the benefits of controllable stress versus uncontrollable stress. When you master or overcome a stressful situation, you gain confidence in your ability to deal with future stress and are less likely to see your stress as overwhelming. If you can feel a sense of control in the midst of a stressful situation, your prefrontal cortex will calm down your amygdala. This doesn't mean you have to control every aspect of the situation or even the final result. You just have to focus your attention on the controllable aspects of your stressor or find some aspect of your life that gives you a sense of accomplishment, despite the ongoing stress. Seeing yourself as someone who has overcome stress and adversity in the past or who has the skills to manage the situation is another way to get your stress levels under control.

CHAPTER 6

Learning Self-Compassion

When you get stressed and your amygdala sends your brain and body into "fight, flight, or freeze" mode, you may experience a sense of urgency or pressure to act. You may pressure yourself to work harder, go faster, and not take breaks. You may constantly be thinking *I'm not doing enough!* and berate yourself for not having enough self-discipline and willpower. Although it's important to try to meet deadlines and solve problems, this sense of pressure can lead you to be too hard on yourself. Never letting up or giving yourself a break can turn acute stress (such as when you're facing a work deadline) into chronic stress. Your brain takes the stress with you wherever you go, which means your body experiences ongoing surges of stress hormones that can exhaust it.

This chapter will show you a different way to motivate yourself in the face of stress. Rather than berating and depriving yourself, you can react with self-compassion. By being more patient, kind, and compassionate with yourself, you can calm down your amygdala and quell your sense of panic. You'll still be motivated to get important things done, but you're likely to be happier and less anxious while doing them.

We Pressure Ourselves When Under Stress

When you face a stressor with important consequences, your amygdala goes into overdrive to make sure that you get the job done.

Although this may seem like a good thing, being too hard on ourselves can be counterproductive. When our ancestors were in the jungle, after they escaped a threat they went back to cooking their food, collecting berries, resting, or finding a mate. Physiologically, their cortisol levels soared when their stress was acute, then quickly dipped down again. Today, we face a different reality. Most of the stresses we face are complex and chronic situations that can go on for years or even decades. Working and worrying all the time will wear you out if you don't also take time to replenish. Constantly berating yourself for not doing enough will just make you more stressed. Although you may get more stuff done, you'll tax your health and your self-esteem.

Most of life's stressors are more like marathons than sprints. If we give it everything we've got in the first mile, how are we going to get through the other twenty-five? In today's world, we're dealing with new stresses coming at us, even as we try to find our way through a chronic situation. You may be dealing with a new baby when an urgent situation comes up at work. Or getting into a fight with your partner when you're trying to figure out how to pay the bills. Or finding out that a loved one has cancer as you're making home repairs. So it doesn't make sense to put all of your energy into dealing with one type of stress—you need to keep reserves on hand for the unexpected crisis that will inevitably rear its head. Physiologically, when stressors are layered on each other without time for recovery, your body's cortisol response can get out of whack, making you more vulnerable to colds and flu, high blood pressure, and inflammatory responses. So take a step back, give yourself a break, and allow yourself just to do what's most important and allow time for rest, rather than trying to do everything all the time.

The Costs of Not Letting Up

"Fight, flight, or freeze" mode is a major reason why you pressure and criticize yourself when under stress. Your amygdala is like a fire alarm that won't shut off. When it starts ringing, the resulting adrenaline and cortisol create so much activation that it's difficult to focus and be strategic in approaching your stress. You may feel compelled to work harder, do more, get by with less food and sleep, spend less time with your family and friends, and have less exercise and downtime. But the truth is that our bodies and brains weren't built to be driven like machines, and you'll end up paying a high price in terms of your health, your happiness, and the quality of your relationships. In my clinical practice, I see many couples trying to juggle young children and high-powered careers, often without much help because their families live far away. Mostly, they come in for couples therapy because the stress has taken such a toll on their relationship. The following story is a good example of what happens when we're too hard on ourselves under stress.

> Greg and Stacey were in their late thirties. Married for four years, they had a nine-month-old daughter and a three-year-old son, and they lived in a house that they were busy renovating. Their families lived far away, and so they had to pay babysitters or swap with friends if they wanted time away from the kids. Money was scarce, because they had a huge mortgage. Greg worked for a biotech start-up that was understaffed and running out of funding, so he was doing the job of three people and under intense pressure. Stacey had her own consulting business and took care of the kids.
>
> The couple's fights and lack of intimacy led them to seek therapy. At their first session, they both told the therapist that ongoing stress was a fact of life for them. Stacey had been prescribed a tranquilizer because she suffered from chronic anxiety. She also used emotional eating to comfort herself. Greg had a fifty-minute commute to work—longer if there was an accident on the freeway. He said he had difficulty sleeping and that he couldn't go back to sleep after Stacey got up at night to feed the baby.

As the session went on, the therapist became aware of how hard both Greg and Stacey were on themselves. Stacey was always feeling guilty because she didn't think she spent enough time with the kids, although in truth she spent almost every waking moment with them when she wasn't working or dealing with contractors. She was constantly multitasking, with a baby in one hand, a toddler in the other, and a cell phone tucked under her neck. Greg felt guilty that Stacey had to bear the brunt of the household stressors because he left home at six in the morning and didn't get home until eight at night. He said he'd like to go to the gym but didn't feel entitled to do so, because it would reduce his time with his family. Each day after Greg came home and after the family ate a quick dinner, both Greg and Stacey would get back on their computers, tag-teaming looking after the kids. By ten o'clock, when the kids were finally asleep, the couple would talk about household and renovation logistics but the conversation would degenerate into fighting, leading both to feel misunderstood and unappreciated. Physical and emotional intimacy were almost nonexistent, because one of them inevitably ended up passing out on the couch at the end of the night. Stacey said she felt like a failure for not being a more thin, sexy, and entertaining wife to her husband and not cooking a healthy meal every night. Greg beat himself up for not earning more, which would have provided more money for babysitters and allowed them to pay down the mortgage.

Greg and Stacey were perfectionists. They had worked extremely hard to get into competitive colleges and succeed as entrepreneurs. They were used to doing everything the right way—staying healthy; being neat, organized, and on top of things; saving money; and having an ideal relationship. When kids came into the picture, it became simply impossible to do everything perfectly anymore. Yet, rather than adjusting their expectations and giving themselves a break, they continued to expect perfection from themselves and each other, which multiplied their stress and guilt. Perfectionism and unnecessary guilt are a curse disguised as a blessing. They'll keep triggering your amygdala to give you the message that you're not doing enough. In order to have a stress-proof brain, you need to let go of perfectionism and guilt. Use the following self-assessment to find out whether guilt and perfectionism are problems for you.

PRACTICE: Assessing Your Guilt and Perfectionism

Using the following scale, rate how much you agree or disagree with each statement: 1 = completely disagree, 2 = mostly disagree, 3 = somewhat disagree, 4 = neither agree nor disagree, 5 = somewhat agree, 6 = mostly agree, and 7 = completely agree.

1. No matter how hard I work, I always feel as if I could be doing more.

2. There are no excuses for making mistakes.

3. I give my very best in everything that I do.

4. If things aren't done perfectly, it feels as if they're not done at all.

5. I always check and recheck my work.

6. If my house isn't organized and tidy, I can't relax.

7. I don't feel good when I put myself first.

8. Being tired is no excuse for taking a break when there's work to be done.

9. If I'm not working or being productive all the time, I feel lazy.

10. I never feel as if I'm doing enough for the people in my life.

11. I need to look after others before I can take care of my own needs.

12. If I eat out, I feel guilty because I could be saving the money.

13. Even though I spend most of my time with my kids or working, I feel I need to do more.

14. I feel guilty complaining about my stress, because others have it worse.

Statements 1–7 indicate perfectionism, whereas statements 8–14 indicate guilt. If you mostly agree or completely agree with more than one or two statements from either group, perfectionism or guilt may be a problem for you.

Perfectionism and guilt add a layer of unnecessary stress to an already stressful situation. Rather than calming your amygdala down, they rile it up. Are you your own biggest critic? Is nothing you do ever good enough to meet your own standards? Perfectionism can result from a rigid mind-set in which you don't adjust your expectations to fit the situation. Think of Greg and Stacey, who wanted to be the perfect parents and partners but ended up just feeling stressed and bad about themselves. Perfectionists have *conditional* self-esteem, meaning they can only like themselves when they do well. But under stressful conditions, we need to adjust our standards and expectations. Sometimes, when we face a barrage of challenges, just surviving is doing well. Perfectionists often feel like impostors or frauds and live in constant fear of being exposed as incompetent. That may be why they're so self-critical and hard-driving. Stressful circumstances can make perfectionism worse, as we struggle to keep our heads above water.

Although perfectionism is an attempt to manage stress by staying in control, it often backfires. Perfectionism can lead to second-guessing, procrastinating, feeling overwhelmed, or giving up and not trying. It can also be dangerous to your mind and body: An article in the *Review of General Psychology* (Flett, Hewitt, and Heisel 2014) tells us that perfectionists are more likely to struggle with depression or anxiety and more likely to commit suicide. Perfectionists are also more likely to be diagnosed with chronic fatigue syndrome or chronic pain.

Just as perfectionism is unhelpful under conditions of stress, so is guilt. Guilt is an emotion we often learn in childhood, when our caregivers say things like "Eat all your food; there are people starving in India" and "I've been working my fingers to the bone to take care of you, and all you do is complain?" As adults, we internalize these messages and feel as if we can never do enough. Stress can trigger feelings of guilt because there's not enough time to get everything done. We may have to choose between meeting our own goals or doing things for others. It becomes more challenging to exercise and live healthy. Other kinds of stressors, such as ending a relationship or having to step away from someone who's toxic to us, can make us feel guilty because someone else may be upset with our decision.

Our culture sends us strong messages about not being selfish and self-indulgent. Unfortunately, people get confused and interpret these messages in an "all or nothing" way. If you lied to someone you care about, or acted in a selfish and hurtful way, then feeling guilt can motivate you to stop the hurtful behavior and make amends (Cryder, Springer, and Morewedge 2012). This will likely improve your relationships and your self-esteem. Many other types of guilt are likely to be counterproductive and make you feel more stressed. When you're stressed, you certainly don't need the additional burden of unnecessary guilt!

To overcome perfectionism and unnecessary guilt, you need to learn new ways of thinking and behaving.

PRACTICES: Ten Ways to Overcome Guilt and Perfectionism

The following practices can help you get started building new habits and brain pathways. Learning new ways of doing things is often challenging and takes time. So be patient with yourself and with the process. It takes months, not days, to really change your brain.

1. If you feel guilty because you're not doing enough for your kids, partner, or family, list all the things that you regularly do for them. Then make another list, of all the things you do to take care of yourself when you're stressed. Which list is longer? If the "do for others" list is as long as or longer than the "do for myself" list, take this as objective proof that you are doing enough for others and don't have reason to feel guilty. If the "do for myself" list is longer, think about whether the self-care activities help you be a better parent, partner, or family member. If they do, then you still have no reason to feel guilty.

2. Instead of feeling guilty, take a direct approach to the problem. Ask the people you think you're neglecting whether they actually feel neglected. Consider whether they have a tendency to expect too much and not take enough responsibility for themselves. Then think about how an outside observer would view the situation. If you conclude that you really aren't doing enough, then sit down with the other person and try to come up with some solutions or compromises that balance everyone's needs.

3. Write a "self-gratitude" diary at the end of every day, noting at least three things you did that day that furthered your goals or helped someone you care about. At the end of the week, read what you've written. Guilt and perfectionism have a negative bias. They make you pay attention to what you're *not* doing right. By writing down what you actually did, you can overcome this bias and force yourself to focus on your accomplishments.

4. To combat guilt, think about how you'd feel if the tables were turned. Put yourself in the other person's shoes. Would you think that the other person wasn't doing enough to help you or meet your needs, given how much he or she has going on? We often find it easy to be compassionate and understanding with others but are too harsh on ourselves. By deliberately taking an "observer" perspective, you'll likely see your situation in a new light.

5. If you're a perfectionist, begin setting limits with yourself. Give yourself a set amount of time to work on each task (whether cleaning the house, planning a party, writing a paper, or completing a work assignment). Don't work for more than forty-five minutes without taking a break to stretch or sit down. Set an alarm to give you a ten-minute warning at the end of the planned time frame. Force yourself to get up and move on to the next task, even if you're not finished. At the end of the day, you can schedule a "catch-up" hour for high-priority tasks that you didn't finish. Notice how much more efficiently you work when you don't allow yourself to take all day.

6. Don't allow yourself to proofread or check your work more than once. Stop reading and rereading that e-mail, trying to come up with the perfect response. It's just not worth it! The same goes for cleaning—after one or two wipes, you need to move on to the next area. Notice how much time you save.

7. Many perfectionists overestimate the negative consequences of making a mistake. They assume it'll be a disaster or that they'll lose money, lose their job, or lose their relationships. The antidote to this is to use the behavioral strategy of "exposure." Decide what mistake you're going to make deliberately. Before you make the mistake, write down what you think will happen as a result. Then notice what actually happens, and compare this to your prediction. Were the consequences as dire as you predicted? If not, what does that teach you?

8. If you're procrastinating because you don't think you'll do a good enough job, just get started. If you want to write a book, set yourself a small goal, such as writing one page every day. Or write without worrying about spelling or grammar. When you've finished your goal, check in with how you feel and decide whether you want to do more. Once you have something written down or a first draft, it's much easier to keep going. Or you can do what my friend did when she was writing her doctoral thesis. She woke up an hour earlier than usual, got a cup of coffee, and wrote while in her pajamas before she had time to realize that she didn't feel like doing it!

9. When you evaluate your own work, take a step back and imagine someone you love, such as your grandma, best friend, or favorite teacher. What would that person say about your efforts? Then switch roles and imagine what you'd think and say if that person had done this work. By looking at your own work through "loving eyes," you can learn to tone down your rigid standards and self-criticism.

10. If you feel self-critical, notice if you're thinking about the situation in a "black and white" way. Perfectionists often see things in all-or-nothing terms: if it's not the best, it must be the worst. Try to find the gray. Consider other ways of seeing the situation. Factor in the situational constraints and barriers you faced; given these challenges, how well did you do? Try to judge your efforts in context, rather than always expecting perfection.

Being More Compassionate with Yourself

In the previous section, you learned how to allow yourself a break and combat your self-judging tendencies. Now you'll learn how to use the attitude of self-compassion to calm down your amygdala's automatic "fight, flight, or freeze" response to stress.

The notion of self-compassion has its roots in Buddhist teachings (Brach 2003; Kornfield 1993; Salzberg 2002). More recently, Kristin Neff, a researcher at the University of Texas, pioneered research into self-compassion as a tool for promoting well-being and stress reduction (Neff 2011). She contrasts self-compassion with self-esteem. Unlike self-esteem, self-compassion doesn't require us to elevate ourselves above other people and compete with them. Whereas high self-esteem is generally based on evidence of superior achievement, self-compassion is a more constant personal quality, in which we value ourselves and treat ourselves kindly just because we're human. This caring attitude toward ourselves helps us recognize our similarity to and connection with other humans. We all have common aspirations and common sources of suffering.

Self-compassion is like Mindfulness Plus. Being mindful means gently noticing what you're thinking, feeling, and doing right now, rather than operating on automatic pilot. It involves asking "Is this what you want to be thinking and doing, or do you need to take a step back?" According to psychologist Christopher Germer (2009), self-compassion expands on this by asking "What is it that you need?" Unmet needs for rest, enjoyment, peace, companionship, acknowledgment, comfort, meaning, money, food, or sex create emotional suffering that interferes with our ability to be goal-oriented. Self-compassion acknowledges these needs, and it encourages us to take care of them in active ways so that they're less likely to interfere with our efforts to manage stress.

In addition to mindfulness, there are two other aspects of self-compassion: self-kindness and common humanity. Self-kindness means being kinder and gentler with yourself—extending the same compassion to yourself that you would to any being that was stressed or suffering. You may find it easy to be understanding and forgiving of others yet beat yourself up for feeling stressed, for not meeting your goals, or for past decisions that got you into this stressful situation. You may even beat yourself up for random events or for other people's bad behavior. Self-kindness makes you take a step back and see your stressful situation and coping efforts in a more compassionate light. Everybody messes up sometimes. You don't have to be perfect; you just have to be human. This attitude can help relieve your feelings of stress, anxiety, and self-criticism.

The most common reason people give for not being more compassionate with themselves is that they don't want to be self-indulgent or wimpy. But this is a faulty assumption. Self-compassion does not make you spoiled or weak but is a learned coping strategy that can decrease anxiety and enhance resilience and recovery from stress. It doesn't require you to be Pollyannaish and deny or suppress negative aspects of your experience. In fact, part of Dr. Neff's definition of self-compassion is mindfulness. Mindfulness helps you stop and notice your feelings of stress and self-critical thoughts, while self-compassion teaches you how to generate feelings of warmth and care toward yourself and, by extension, toward others who are stressed or suffering.

A recent meta-analysis (MacBeth and Gumley 2012) statistically combined the results of twenty studies exploring links between self-compassion and psychopathology. Results indicated that self-compassion was reliably and strongly associated with less depression, less anxiety, and less stress. Feeling compassion toward yourself decreases stress and anxiety in evaluative situations, such as when you're being asked about your weaknesses in a job interview (Neff, Kirkpatrick, and Rude 2007). Self-compassion is also associated with higher and more consistent levels of well-being than self-esteem (Neff and Vonk 2009). Our self-esteem often varies depending on the situation: we feel good when we're doing well, but not so good when we fail or make mistakes; we're only as good as our last accomplishment. With self-compassion, our self-evaluations aren't dependent on constant proof of achievement, so we can we feel more relaxed and better about our lives, even with ongoing stress. Self-compassion is also associated with more curiosity and exploration. When we don't beat ourselves up for failure, we're freer to try new things and make mistakes as part of our learning and growth. People who are self-compassionate are also more willing to take responsibility for their part when things don't turn out as planned. When you don't see mistakes as proof of your deficiency, this frees you to admit to your mistakes, apologize, get feedback, and make amends, rather than hide away in shame. Self-compassion is a powerful tool that helps you learn from stress!

Self-compassion may help people overcome emotional eating, which is a very common response to stress. In one study of restricted and guilty eaters (Adams and Leary 2007), students were given doughnuts to eat, but half of the students were assigned at random to hear a compassionate comment from the experimenter, such as "Don't beat yourself up about eating these; subjects eat them all the time." The other half received the doughnuts without the comment. Later that day, when given the chance to eat candy, those who had heard the compassionate comment ate less. Ironically, harsh self-criticism seems to create an inner rebelliousness that makes us want to give up on our healthy goals. Self-compassion acknowledges the reality that it's an unhealthy moment, not an unhealthy life, and you have a choice what the next moment is going to be. And it motivates you to make a healthy, compassionate choice.

Research shows that self-compassion can help us adapt to major life events, disappointments, and chronic stressors. One study (Sbarra, Smith, and Mehl 2012) found that self-compassion was essential in helping people adjust to life after divorce. Another study linked self-compassion to greater resilience and reduced avoidance in dealing with academic failure (Neff, Hsieh, and Dejitterat 2005). In a third study, people coping with chronic pain who were higher in self-compassion were less likely to view their situation as a catastrophe and were less disabled by the pain than those who were less self-compassionate (Wren et al. 2012).

When you face highly stressful situations or losses, your natural tendency might be to ask yourself what you did wrong. Saying to yourself instead, *I did the best I could given what I knew at the time*, can help you feel better and give you more courage to face your stressors and persist when things get tough.

On a physiological level, self-compassion is like a soothing balm to your amygdala. It sends the message to your brain that you're not under imminent threat and don't have to use an emergency response. Rather, you can take your time, relax, and give your prefrontal cortex time to respond. As a result, your amygdala sends a signal to terminate the stress response and turn off the flow of excess cortisol. Even if a situation is stressful, you don't have to make it more stressful for yourself by making your self-esteem dependent on performing perfectly. Rather, you can learn to feel good about yourself just for trying your best. When circumstances are extremely difficult, you need to give yourself credit merely for surviving. This maxim applies to unemployment, financial stress, divorce, keeping a company going in stressful times, difficult office politics, learning that a loved one has a serious illness, and many other stressful situations.

Practicing self-compassion over months or years can build new pathways in your brain. Rather than compounding your stress by worrying, blaming, or criticizing yourself, you can calm down your amygdala by treating yourself with kindness and understanding. Think of it this way: When a child starts crying, what might a good parent do? The parent might pick up the child, speak soothingly, and guide the child gently to solve the problem. With self-compassion, you become a good parent to yourself. When you mess up or have a bad day, you gently get yourself back on track. This approach is helpful in overcoming addiction and sticking to healthy-living plans as well as managing stress.

One way to enhance your self-compassion is through meditation. Loving-kindness meditation, or *metta*, is a Buddhist teaching to develop qualities of altruistic love. The word *metta* is an ancient Pali (Buddhist) term denoting loving-kindness, friendliness, benevolence, and nonviolence. It expresses a strong wish for the well-being and happiness of others. Meditation teacher Sharon Salzberg interprets the Buddha's teachings as meaning that we need to learn to love ourselves in order to love others. She paraphrases the Buddha's teachings as saying that "You yourself, as much as anybody in the entire universe, deserve your love and affection" (Salzberg 2002, 31). Therefore, *metta* has components that direct love and kindness to the self as well. In the following version of *metta*, which I constructed based on meditations by Sharon Salzberg (2002) and others, you wish yourself and others relief from stress. Other versions of *metta* involve directing kind and loving thoughts and well wishes toward different types of people.

PRACTICE: Loving-Kindness Meditation

Sit quietly with your legs crossed, and maintain an upright and relaxed pose. Begin to notice your breathing, and let your mind and body settle. Take a few slow breaths—noticing your inhalations and exhalations. Now think about the stress you're facing. Try to get a visual image of your stressed self. What do you feel in your body? What thoughts fill your mind? What's the expression on your face? Imagine yourself rushing around or worrying. As you contemplate this image, become aware of the suffering that the stress is causing you, and become aware of your deep wish to be at ease and at peace. Now think about somebody past or present, real or imaginary, who loves and cares about you deeply. Imagine this person looking at you with deep caring and compassion. And imagine him or her saying the following to you:

"Dear (insert your name here),

"I see how stressed and tired you are. How much you suffer with your feelings of stress. How anxious and overwhelmed you feel. And I send these wishes to you:

"May you be healthy.

"May you be safe and secure.

"May you be at peace with yourself and others.

"May you live with ease and happiness."

After saying this a few times, bid farewell to your loved one.

Now imagine saying these same words to yourself. Say them a few times, and notice how it feels to hear these kind wishes expressed toward you. If you feel any discomfort or self-consciousness, let those feelings be there. Notice any resistance you have to wishing yourself well. As you keep practicing *metta*, the resistance will lessen. It's not important that you believe the words right now. It's just important that you say them.

Once you're more comfortable expressing *metta* to yourself, you can extend it to include:

- Your family members who are also affected by your stress

- Your friends and colleagues who face the stress with you

- Difficult people in your life who cause stress for you

- All living beings who deal with stress and suffering

Remember to bring up a visual image of each person or group prior to saying the phrases. Notice these people in their state of stress and then send them loving-kindness. You may have difficulty wishing *metta* to people who seem to be the source of your stress. But if they didn't suffer as much and were more at ease, they would cause less stress for you! And if they grew from the experience, they might act in a more mature way and be less stressful to deal with. If you can't yet wish them well out of compassion or tolerance for them, it's okay to send *metta* to them for these "selfish" reasons.

Metta is a practice that gets more powerful over time. Try to practice it regularly at the same time each day, such as when you first wake up or before you go to sleep. Notice any changes in how stressed you feel and whether you feel an internal softening.

The next practice, which I designed, combines aspects of schema therapy imagery practices (Young, Klosko, and Weishaar 2003) and compassion practices (Gilbert 2010) to help you become a loving advocate for yourself. In it, you'll ask your inner critic to step aside and make room for a more compassionate presence.

PRACTICE: Asking the Critic to Step Aside

You can do this practice (1) by deliberately imagining your inner critic and thinking about what it would say to you or (2) whenever you find yourself being self-critical. Most people close their eyes during this practice, in order to be more present with the images.

Listen to your inner critic for a moment. What judgmental and critical things do you hear? Perhaps that you're a loser or not competent, that you've made a mess of your life, or that you're going to fail. Just listen to the words, and notice how they make you feel. How does it feel to hear these unkind words when you're feeling stressed and trying to do your best? Notice how you feel in your body.

Now put a face to this critical voice. Perhaps it's the face of one of your parents, teachers, coaches, or romantic partners who used to speak to you in this way. Or it might be the face of an imaginary being, such as a witch, or an animal, such as a wolf or an alligator. Whatever it looks like is okay. Picture the critic standing there berating you.

Now bring into the image a wise person or being who cares deeply about you. It can be someone from your past or present, a spiritual figure (such as Jesus or the Buddha), or an imaginary creature. It may be someone you knew well or someone you didn't know well but whom you know is a good person. It can even be a character from a book, a movie, or TV, such as Superman or Oprah Winfrey. Imagine that this being, seeing you listening to your inner critic, is filled with love and compassion for you. Imagine the compassionate being stepping between you and the critic and holding up a hand, telling the critic kindly but firmly to stop. Picture the compassionate being telling the critic that the way it's behaving is hurting you or causing you stress and it needs to say what it needs to say with kindness. Imagine the critic saying what it's really afraid of—or just quieting down—and then moving to one side, leaving you with your compassionate being. Now imagine the compassionate being comforting you with physical gestures and kind, encouraging words. Imagine him or her giving you a hug or taking your hand, giving you a high five, and so on. Imagine what words of encouragement he or she might say to you. Maybe something like "You'll get through this and succeed. Just keep trying." Notice what you feel in your mind and body as you feel the compassion and words of encouragement. You may feel a bit teary-eyed or notice yourself softening. Perhaps nobody has stood up for you and encouraged you like this before. Now you'll always have this inner compassionate being to protect and support you. Imagine the compassionate being becoming a part of you. And when you're ready, open your eyes and come back to the room.

Final Thoughts

In this chapter, you learned how guilt and perfectionism can increase your stress and how to overcome these tendencies. You learned that self-compassion is a coping strategy for stress and an attitude toward life. Having self-compassion means being kind to yourself and realizing you're only human, so you don't have to be perfect. It involves connecting with the unmet needs that underlie your stressed-out behavior. You can increase your self-compassion by speaking kindly to yourself and giving yourself a break or through loving-kindness meditation and imagery.

PART 3

Moving Forward with Your Prefrontal Cortex

CHAPTER 7

Becoming Cognitively Flexible

In part 2 of this book, you learned strategies for calming your amygdala's rapid automatic "fight, flight, or freeze" response to a stressor. In the remainder of the book, you'll learn stress-reducing strategies based on your prefrontal cortex's logical thinking capacities. Your prefrontal cortex integrates information from past experience to modify your amygdala's perceptions of threat. It also helps you inhibit destructive responses, such as addictive or aggressive tendencies. Your prefrontal cortex helps you benefit from past learning, so that you can get better at managing stressors over time.

This system works well if your past experiences and environment provided you with enough guidance and support to teach you how to cope effectively with stressors. However, perhaps your parents modeled or taught you unhelpful responses to stress, such as worrying all the time, overworking, drinking too much alcohol, pretending the stressor wasn't happening, or being hostile and distrusting. Perhaps they didn't give you enough guidance and emotional support because they were always working, were depressed, were ill, or didn't understand the responsibilities of a good parent. Or perhaps they were overprotective and didn't let you make decisions or try to solve problems on your own. In these cases, your experiences may have led you to faulty or unrealistic assumptions about how the world works or to stick rigidly to one way of reacting, without realizing that you need a whole toolbox of coping strategies for different situations.

Integrated and Unintegrated Brain Responses to Stress

Daniel Siegel, a psychiatrist and pioneer of interpersonal neurobiology (the science of how our brains and minds relate to ourselves and other people), claims that the pathways between our brain neurons form as a result of the way our caretakers relate to us (Siegel 2010). Children who are nurtured and understood by their caretakers develop the ability to understand their own feelings and communicate those feelings. They also implicitly learn that their feelings are valid, and so they develop trust in themselves and their own judgment, rather than having to second-guess themselves all the time. Children who receive empathy and guidance from caretakers are better able to soothe their own emotions and set limits with themselves, rather than feeling as if the world will end if they don't get what they want (whether it's a candy or a promotion).

In brain terms, adults who, as children, experienced secure attachment with a caregiver have more well-developed prefrontal cortices and more integrated brain networks. In other words, secure attachment facilitates a brain network in which there are clearer pathways linking the prefrontal cortex to the amygdala, the hippocampus, and other structures so that information flows freely between these areas. On the other hand, children who didn't experience this secure attachment have less integrated brains. Unless this deficiency has been repaired by later relationships, they're less likely to come up with effective, creative responses to stress that take into account their thoughts, their feelings, their personal history, other people's reactions, the resources available to them, and the demands of the situation as it unfolds.

If you didn't have good childhood attachment experiences, you can still develop a more integrated brain as an adult if you have close friends, partners, or even therapists and coaches who provide you with emotional support, help you understand yourself better, and model healthy ways of reacting to stress. You can also begin to grow a stress-proof brain, even as an adult, if you keep practicing the strategies in this book. Mindfulness alone has been shown to beneficially affect the functioning of eight different brain areas involved in self-control, self-awareness, and emotion regulation. These are all skills that can help you cope more effectively with stress. It may take a few months for your brain to begin changing, so stick with it!

When your brain has integrated neuronal networks as a result of secure attachment or adult learning, information can flow rapidly back and forth between your amygdala, hippocampus, and prefrontal cortex and between the two hemispheres of your brain. As mentioned in chapter 1, your brain has two hemispheres, one on each side. Your right hemisphere processes information in a global, holistic way and is more spatial, emotional, and creative. Your left hemisphere, on the other hand, tends to be logical, linear, factual, and verbal. In general, positive emotion is represented more in the left hemisphere and negative emotion in the right. Although this is a bit of an oversimplification, it's helpful for our purposes.

Those of us with less well-connected brains have a less integrated and coordinated response to stress. We may focus only on left-hemisphere logical thinking while ignoring our emotional response to the stressor. When we feel stressed, we may try to fix the problem right away without giving ourselves the opportunity to understand how we feel and what we need. Eventually, our coping responses may break down, or we may experience an unsatisfactory outcome because of unmet emotional needs that we haven't acknowledged. Another type of cognitive rigidity is too much persistence—we may persist in looking at the stressful situation in the same way and using the same strategies we always have, regardless of whether they're actually working in this situation. For example, we may put in huge amounts of unsuccessful effort to fix things when the stress is caused by somebody else's issues.

Betty was facing chronic stress in her marriage. Her husband seemed to always be dissatisfied and critical of her, and this affected her self-esteem. He would criticize her weight, appearance, competence, and personality. Betty had grown up with a critical father, so she responded to the marital stress by doing what she always did—trying harder to please, dieting obsessively (although she wasn't really overweight), or spending her whole day cleaning, cooking, and organizing the house, without ever doing anything fun for herself. She began to feel depressed when her husband's behavior didn't change despite her best efforts.

After getting therapy, Betty finally realized that her husband was the problem. He had unrealistic expectations and was critical and intolerant. The best response to the situation was not to try harder but to ask her husband to change his behavior or leave the relationship. Because as a child, Betty had learned to placate her abusive father in order to avoid his anger, she was initially able to view the problem with her husband only through the lens of her own "badness," and the only response she knew was to keep trying harder, even if her efforts clearly weren't working. Therapy taught her to be more cognitively flexible and view the problem in a different way, which led to a more functional coping strategy: she decided to leave the marriage.

Another type of unintegrated brain response to stress is emotional chaos. This is when your brain reacts only from the right hemisphere, with emotional stress and feelings of panic. Because your logical left brain capacities are offline, you may feel overwhelmed and helpless—unable to focus and think clearly or take steps to address the problem. At another level, your prefrontal cortex may not be communicating effectively with your amygdala, making you unable to shut off "fight, flight, or freeze" mode. You continue to react with responses appropriate to an emergency. Also, because your right hemisphere is linked to negative emotions, you may see the situation in an overly pessimistic light, making you feel depressed and helpless. This type of chaotic reaction is more common in people who have had abusive or neglectful childhoods. Chaotic reactions feel overwhelming, because you literally can't use your prefrontal cortex to think clearly or see the situation realistically. If you have this type of response, you may be more likely to feel panicky or to resort to avoidance and addictive behaviors to soothe the overwhelming feelings.

Peggy was an administrative assistant working in a financial services company. The workload was very high, and her bosses were demanding and critical. Peggy was in her late thirties and lived alone, with no family members nearby. She was under constant financial stress because of increasing rents, having an old car, and not having any family to fall back on in case of a crisis. She hated her job and knew she should try to find another one, but she couldn't motivate herself to update her résumé and write cover letters. She felt lonely, but she didn't try to meet friends or potential partners because she felt so undesirable and overweight. She was behind on deadlines at work, but when she came home in the evening, she felt too overwhelmed to do anything. She would turn on the TV, open a bottle of wine and a box of cookies, and stay on the couch for the rest of the evening.

Eventually Peggy sought psychotherapy. She learned to use mindfulness to calm down her inner panic enough to focus. As a result of worrying less, Peggy had more energy and willpower left over at the end of the day. Through therapy, she learned that she wasn't helpless and had, in fact, survived a very abusive childhood without much help from anyone. She learned how to challenge her negative thinking and began taking steps to solve her problems. Eventually, she found a more satisfying job, lost twenty pounds, and entered into a relationship.

Both Betty (described earlier) and Peggy initially had unintegrated brain responses to stress. Betty's was rigid, whereas Peggy's was chaotic and avoidant. Through therapy, both Betty and Peggy learned to view their stressful situations in a different light, which opened the door for more effective coping options. They both learned how to inhibit their habitual, ineffective coping responses and try new ways of coping. In brain terms, you could say that they learned the skill of cognitive flexibility.

Cognitive flexibility involves the ability to consider conflicting information (for example, Peggy's job provided some financial security but also involved unhealthy stress) and to adjust your responses based on changes in the situation as it unfolds. For example, if Betty's husband had responded to her expressions of dissatisfaction in a positive, loving way and tried to become less critical, it might have made sense to change her plan to leave the marriage.

Stress and Cognitive Flexibility

Cognitive flexibility is an essential skill in successfully negotiating stress. Think of cognitive flexibility as working with mental clay; you can mold your brain in different ways until you find a way of thinking and coping that best fits the situation. Cognitive rigidity, by comparison, is like working with cement, and cognitive chaos is like working with sand.

Stress may automatically decrease your cognitive flexibility and narrow your perspective. Stress makes you cling to old habits and be less likely to explore new options. This can even happen in infants! In one study (Seehagen et al. 2015), 26 fifteen-month-old infants participated in a learning task. The infants who had already been exposed to stressful situations in the lab, such as a stranger sitting down next to them or their parents leaving the room for a few minutes, showed an increase in cortisol during the task. The infants in the control group, who hadn't been exposed to stress, didn't show increased cortisol. Then both groups were given lamps that gave off either a red light or a blue light when pressed. The infants were allowed to press only one of the lamps as often as they liked. In the next part of the experiment, the infants could choose which lamp to play with, but now neither lamp lit up. Even though the lamps no longer worked, infants in the stress condition continued to press the lamp that they were originally given. Children in the control group pressed the other lamp significantly more frequently, showing more flexible behavior.

If stress causes infants as young as fifteen months to stick to old habits, it's no wonder that those of us who have experienced stressful childhoods are more likely to keep doing the same old thing when we feel stressed. Stress and anxiety narrow our focus, making threats seem larger than they really are. This "tunnel vision" makes it likely we'll overreact using habitual strategies that may not be appropriate for the situation. The following practice will teach you to be more cognitively flexible and take different perspectives on a stressful situation.

PRACTICE: Learning Cognitive Flexibility

Think about a stressful situation that you're currently facing. In a journal or on a separate piece of paper, write a brief (two or three lines) description of your situation. Now think about the way you see this situation. Do you see it as a threat, a challenge, a loss, or all of the above? If you're seeing it as a threat or loss, is there any way to see it as a challenge? What do you have to lose, or what do you have to learn? What are your priorities and goals in dealing with this situation?

How controllable do you think the situation is? If it's a changing situation or one with an uncertain outcome, write down some ways it may change over time or some possible outcomes. Do you need to modify your view of the situation, priorities, or goals to deal with these potential changes?

How have you been coping with this situation? Is this the same way that you typically cope with stress? How well is it working for you? What are the pros and cons of using this approach? Is it helping you feel better? Is it solving the problem?

How successful has this strategy been for you in the past? Is the current situation similar to what you've faced in the past, or are there differences? If there are differences, do you need to adjust your strategy? If you're using a strategy that hasn't been successful in the past, think about why you're still using it. What's keeping you from trying something new?

Now think about other people involved in the situation (including the person you're having conflict with, if appropriate). What's their view of the situation? Do they see it as a threat, a challenge, or a loss? What are their most pressing priorities and goals? Is there anything you can do to reach a compromise or work together with these people, or do you need to set better boundaries for yourself?

Now try to find the most objective viewpoint. How might neutral observers see the situation? How might they see your role in the stressor? What do they see you doing that is helping or hurting? How might they see the other people's roles and contribution?

Think about someone you know who copes well with stress, or someone you admire. How might this person see this situation? Would this person see it as a threat, a challenge, a loss, or all three? What would this person's most important goals and priorities be? How would this person cope with the stressful situation?

Is there anything you can learn from considering these different viewpoints? Are there any new perspectives or strategies that might be helpful to you? How might you implement them? Are there any internal or external barriers that you need to overcome?

Overcoming Worry and Rumination

Now that you have some tools for overcoming mental rigidity or chaos, let's talk about two other common but unproductive responses to stress—worry and rumination.

Worry "represents an attempt to engage in mental problem-solving on an issue whose outcome is uncertain but contains the possibility of one or more negative outcomes; consequently worry relates closely to the fear process" (Borkovec et al. 1983, 10).

Research on worry suggests that it may reduce physiological arousal and negative images by keeping you in the verbal realm (Borkovec and Hu 1990). Worry is left-brain focused and may keep you focused on the details, preventing you from seeing the big picture. Some researchers (Borkovec, Alcaine, and Behar 2004) think that worrying may be a way of avoiding the bodily signs of anxiety and stress (such as your heart beating rapidly) or negative mental images related to your stressor (such as the image of having to sell and move out of your house).

Worry can magnify the stressor by bringing up more and more negative possibilities. One negative thought leads to another, and you start feeling more and more stressed. Worry makes you feel as if the worst is already happening (our brains don't always distinguish between imagination and reality). Short-term worry can be productive if it helps you plan and solve problems. Worry can also be helpful if it leads to new perspectives on the problem. But often worry turns into rumination.

Rumination is persistent and repetitive worry, in which you revisit the same information repeatedly without finding any new answers. Rumination goes beyond trying to solve a problem or deal with a stressor. Your thoughts go from *What negative outcomes are likely to happen and how could I prevent them?* to things like *Why am I such a loser? Why did I make such poor decisions that led to this situation? Why can't I cope? What's going to happen if I keep feeling stressed like this?* The word "rumination" describes what a cow does when "chewing its cud"—chewing, swallowing, regurgitating, and then chewing it again. In the same way, we mull the same information over and over when we ruminate, without finding new perspectives on our stress.

Worry and rumination are the result of a "feedback loop" between your amygdala and your prefrontal cortex. When your amygdala sends out its alarm signals, your prefrontal cortex analyzes the alarm (worry) and then, instead of calming down your amygdala, comes up with other things that might go wrong. This creates a vicious cycle of escalating and self-perpetuating alarm and worry between your amygdala and your prefrontal cortex. Research using brain scans shows that rumination is associated with increased amygdala activity during the processing of emotional stimuli (Siegle, Ingram, and Matt 2002).

Rumination is also associated with increased depression and anxiety over time (Nolen-Hoeksema 2000). If you ruminate when you're feeling down about a problem, you're likely to feel even worse. Ruminators want to understand why the stressor is happening and its meaning for their lives, but they often end up focusing on the past and blaming and criticizing themselves in unhelpful ways. Ruminators may come up with ways to combat stress (such as work harder or do more exercise), but they're less likely to actually implement these solutions. Rumination can bring up feelings of shame that make you want to hide and run away, rather than dealing actively with the stressor. When people ruminate, they're likely to drink more alcohol or binge to take their focus away from the shame and self-criticism. Rumination can become a thinking trap that justifies avoidance and not taking responsibility for solving the stressful situation or living up to day-to-day responsibilities (such as cleaning the house or taking care of kids) when you're stressed.

Rumination can also have negative consequences for relationships. In a study of bereaved adults (Nolen-Hoeksema and Davis 1999), ruminators were more likely to reach out for social support after their loss, but they reported more friction and that their friends and family gave them less emotional support. Their friends and family members seemed to become frustrated with their ongoing need to talk about their loss and its negative meanings for their lives even many months later. If you keep talking about the same stressful situation over and over, without taking action, people may start viewing you negatively and thinking you should try harder to move on or do something to solve the problem. In one study (Davis et al. 2000), looking for meaning in the loss of a spouse or child was helpful only to the extent that a meaning (such as "It was God's will" or "It was a wake-up call") was actually found. Continuing to look for meaning without finding any just makes you feel more helpless.

When you're stressed, you probably tend to think about the stressor all the time. Your amygdala has a hard time dealing with unresolved problems. It keeps bringing up your stressors and reminding you that you haven't found a solution yet.

PRACTICES: Moving On from Worry and Rumination

It's very difficult to distinguish helpful ways of thinking about your stressors from unhelpful ones. Your brain will try to convince you that you're helping yourself by worrying and ruminating. The following practices can help you break free from rumination.

1. If you find yourself worrying about your stressor, ask yourself how helpful the worry is. Are you actually finding new solutions and making concrete plans to implement them? Are you seeing the situation in a new light or in a more positive way? Do you feel better after thinking about the problem in this way, or do you feel worse? If you aren't finding solutions and new perspectives and you feel worse, then the worry is unhelpful and you need to focus on something else.

2. Practice thought-stopping. Wrap an elastic band around your wrist, and snap it hard every time you notice yourself beginning to worry or ruminate. Shout aloud, "Stop!" (or shout it to yourself if it's not socially appropriate to shout it out). Visualize a big red stop sign. Or visualize a detour sign, directing you onto a new mental track.

3. Make a "worry corner" in your house, or designate a chair as your "worry chair." Allow yourself to worry about your stressor only when you're in your worry chair or corner. Give yourself fifteen minutes two or three times a day to sit and worry. If worries come up at other times, either write them down or save them up for your next worry period. Soon your brain will learn to associate worry only with your worry chair and associate all your other activities with the absence of worry. In this way, you can satisfy your urge to worry in a controlled, time-limited way.

4. Picture your worries as bubbles popping in the air, or as leaves floating down a stream. This is a mindfulness technique that can give you some distance from your worries.

5. Find an alternative, funny image to focus on every time you start worrying. In a classic study of thought suppression (Wegner et al. 1987), participants who were instructed not to think about a white bear ironically couldn't stop themselves from thinking about a white bear. But, when given an alternative image, they could focus on that instead. My favorite image is a bright pink elephant on roller skates. When you start to worry or ruminate, think of your elephant!

6. For one week, notice and record the triggers that make you worry or ruminate (such as talking to another anxious person, lying awake in bed, or watching TV). Now come up with some alternative, positive things to do or ways to avoid those triggers: For example, don't talk about your problems with a person who tends to react negatively or make you more anxious. If you're lying awake worrying at night, get up after fifteen minutes and read a book, listen to music, or watch TV. Schedule fun or distracting activities (going to the gym, walking in nature, doing jigsaws or word puzzles, doing organizational tasks, cooking, going out with friends, talking

to a friend on the phone, and so on) during times that you would normally be ruminating.

7. Interrupt worry cycles by getting up and walking around or by mindfully checking in with what's happening in your body. If you notice an area of tension, send some breaths into that area to open up space or create a bit of softening. Try to give the tension a label, such as "fear," "anger," or "sadness." This can overcome the avoidance associated with being "in your head" and feeling disconnected from your surroundings or your bodily sensations.

De-catastrophizing

Many people catastrophize when under stress. They magnify how bad the stressor is and turn it into a catastrophe that's going to ruin their lives. They also overestimate the likelihood of disastrous events. School shootings, child abductions, airplane crashes, and economic collapses are very bad but very rare occurrences. News editors try to attract viewers or readers by sensationalizing these events so that we pay more attention to them. Most of the things we worry about won't ever happen. Even if they do, we can find ways to cope or to get support. But our brains don't know that, because they're survival-oriented and focused on avoiding a repetition of bad events from our past or negative outcomes we've heard about from the media or other people.

If you've faced an intense and unexpected stressor, such as a car accident, your partner cheating on you, your parents suddenly getting divorced, or your dad losing his job, you may be always on edge, waiting for the other shoe to drop. Your memories of negative events intrude on the present and make you even more reactive to current stressors.

PRACTICE: De-catastrophizing and Probability Estimation

In this practice, which is used in cognitive behavioral therapy for anxiety, you'll learn to calm your amygdala using cognitive strategies from your prefrontal cortex and the (logical, verbal) left side of your brain. Ask yourself the following questions in relation to your current stressor. Write your answers in a journal or on a separate piece of paper.

What am I afraid will happen? (Be very specific—for example, "I'll lose my job" or "My wife will leave me.")

Are these things that will definitely happen or things that might happen? Am I confusing thoughts (which are really guesses about what might happen) *with facts?*

What evidence do I have that these things will happen? Is there any evidence suggesting that they won't happen?

What's the best thing that could happen? Conversely, what's the worst thing that could happen? What's most likely to happen? Why is this outcome most likely?

If the worst did happen, how bad would it be? On a scale of 0 to 100, with 100 being a loved one dying, what would I rate this event?

Could I survive the worst possible outcome? If my family members are likely to be affected, could they survive it? What aspects of my and my family members' life would stay the same, even if it happens? (For example, "We would have to sell our house or leave our neighborhood, but we'd still be able to buy or rent a house in a nearby neighborhood.")

What strategies could I use to cope with the worst possible outcome if it did happen?

If the worst did happen, are there any resources or sources of support I could rely on to help me get through it (friends or family, loans, government programs, and so on)?

Does the stressful event feel less like a catastrophe now? Why, and in what way?

Diagnosing and Overcoming Thinking Traps

In addition to overestimating how bad an event is and underestimating your ability to cope, there are other thinking traps that you can get caught up in when under stress. Stress makes us less cognitively flexible and more likely to see things in "all or nothing" ways. Following are some common thinking traps that may be making you feel worse about your situation.

Black-and-white thinking. Are you seeing things in black and white and forgetting about the gray? This kind of thinking tells you that either things are perfect or they're terrible; you're either a success or a failure—there's nothing in between.

Emotional reasoning. Do you assume something is true just because it *feels* true? For example, you think you're a loser or unlovable because it just feels that way. When you feel down or have been rejected, you're more likely to see yourself and others negatively without any evidence to support your views.

Tunnel vision. Do your feelings about the stressor dominate your life, to the point they're all you can focus on? Do you forget about the aspects of your life that the stressor doesn't affect? When your amygdala sounds the alarm, it focuses your attention narrowly on the stressor. You become preoccupied with planning for something bad or trying to prevent it from happening. You may be extra vigilant for signs that it's already happening. As a result, positive aspects of your life have a lower priority in your brain, which leads to a negative bias.

Wishful thinking. Are you organizing your life around what you hope will happen, rather than preparing for different possible outcomes? Do you not have a backup plan? For example, you're accumulating credit-card debt, hoping you'll earn more money in the future. Or you don't study for an exam and just hope you'll do well. Wishful thinking is a kind of passive coping, in which you don't face the reality of what's actually happening. You feel less stressed in the short term, but your failure to plan can make the stress worse later on. Beneath the wishful thinking, you're probably feeling a great deal of anxiety.

Personalizing. Are you interpreting the stressor too personally and seeing yourself as responsible for it, without any evidence? Often stressors happen because of factors beyond your control. Just because you get cancer doesn't mean you weren't looking after your health. You may be laid off or not find a job because of the state of the economy, not because you're not good enough. Your partner may leave you because he or she has commitment issues, not because of anything you did or didn't do. Personalizing leads you to believe you did something wrong to cause a negative outcome, but that may not be the case.

Blaming yourself or others. Rather than focusing on the current situation and what you can do about it, do you blame yourself for past decisions that didn't work out? Or do you blame other people without taking responsibility for your contribution to the problem? Blame is generally an unhelpful mind-set, because most problems are multifaceted. Blame is also past-focused, rather than present-focused, which makes you hold on to anger and other negative feelings. If you made the best decision you could, given what you knew at the time, then you don't have reason to blame yourself if it didn't work out.

Guilt and regret. Guilt and regret don't do any good unless they can help you change the situation or your behavior in the present. If you've acted against your values or hurt yourself and people you love, guilt can help you make amends. But once you've made amends, you need to forgive yourself. Otherwise guilt will keep you from being mentally present for the people you love. If you're regretting a past decision, are you taking the prior circumstances into account? Hindsight is 20/20. You may know a lot more now than you did then. At the time you made the decision, you may not have had the same information that you have now.

Pessimism. When you think about your stressor, are you seeing the glass as half empty? When you feel stressed, your negative mood may prevent you from seeing the positive or neutral aspects of the situation. Pessimistic thinking makes you feel like giving up because all is lost, but mostly this isn't the case. When you focus on only the negative aspects of a stressful situation, you may start to feel depressed or not see the whole picture accurately.

Overthinking things and second-guessing yourself. Every time you try to make a decision or take a course of action, do you begin to doubt yourself? Do you start thinking of all the negatives or things that could go wrong? Overthinking things and second-guessing yourself can make you feel stuck. Remind yourself that you don't need to wait for the perfect answer before you act.

Unhelpful comparisons. Do you compare yourself to others who seem to be doing better or coping better with stress? Perhaps other people have more money, more energy, more friends, or a better job or house. They may exercise more, eat healthier, or take better care of themselves. Comparing yourself to such people will make you feel worse about yourself and your situation. Know that other people's lives may not be what they seem, whereas your challenges may have created inner strengths you don't fully appreciate.

Judging mind. Do you judge and criticize yourself for not doing what you think you "should" be doing? Or tell yourself you should be doing more, but you don't actually do it? If so, try to understand the real reasons that you're not taking the "perfect" steps to solve the problem.

Getting caught in a thinking trap can increase your stress and create anxiety and depression. Not only are you dealing with a difficult event, but now your own interpretation of why it happened makes you feel bad about yourself. You may get caught in a downward spiral in which negative thoughts and feelings of alarm feed each other. You may feel more helpless to do anything about the stressor. Or you may start to see your life and future in the most negative light.

PRACTICE: Diagnosing Thinking Traps

To alleviate your stress and prevent further damage to your self-esteem, you need to know your thinking traps and label them, rather than continuing to believe what they tell you.

1. Think about a stressful situation you're facing. In a journal or on a separate piece of paper, write a one- or two-paragraph description of the facts of the situation. Facts are things that actually happened or that somebody could observe. They don't include judgments, opinions, or predictions.

2. Write down your personal view of the situation. Why do you think it happened? What implications does it have for your life? What does it say about you and your abilities? What do you want to do about it? What's stopping you from acting? How do you think the situation is going to end? Write down any negative thoughts you have about yourself or others relating to this situation.

3. Read through what you've written, and highlight or underline any parts of it that can be classified as one of the thinking traps we've talked about. Label which thinking trap it is.

PRACTICE: Overcoming Thinking Traps

To overcome thinking traps, try to see the situation in a more positive light. For each thinking trap you identified in the previous practice, ask yourself the following questions:

Black-and-white thinking:

- *Am I thinking in absolutes?*

- *How do I find the gray?*

- *Can I see things from a more balanced perspective?*

- *How can I can be less negative or judgmental?*

- *Is there anything good that can come out of a situation that I'm labeling "all bad"?*

- *Is there a more nuanced way to view the situation?*

- *How might I learn to adjust to the "bad" outcome if it happens?*

Tunnel vision:

- *Am I overemphasizing one piece of the problem and ignoring the big picture?*

- *If I'm just focused on the negative, what positive aspects of my life am I ignoring?*

- *If I'm just seeing my weaknesses, what are my strengths?*

Wishful thinking:

- *Am I focusing on what I wish would happen, rather than what's actually happening?*

- *Based on my past experience and current knowledge, what would I say is most likely to happen, and how can I best plan for it?*

- *What's my backup plan?*

Personalizing:

- *Am I taking things too personally or taking all the responsibility when other people or outside factors contributed to the situation?*

- *What would an objective observer say?*

- *Am I remembering that stress is a universal experience and a natural part of life, rather than a sign that I've messed up?*

Blaming yourself or others:

- *Am I blaming just one person when many different factors contributed?*

- *Am I being too hard on myself or others?*

- *Am I looking at the whole picture and taking the situational factors into account?*

- *How can I focus on dealing with the problem now, rather than blaming?*

Guilt and regret:

- *Did I intentionally hurt anybody or fail to act when I should have?*

- *Did I do what I thought was best, given my capacities and knowledge at the time?*

- *What external factors influenced my decision?*

- *Did I feel frozen, panicked, or overwhelmed?*

- *What past experiences led me to act in this way?*

- *What do I know now that I didn't know then?*

- *How might I begin to let go and forgive myself?*

- *How can I stay focused on dealing with the present, rather than looking back?*

Pessimism:

- *Am I seeing the glass as half empty?*

- *What good parts of my life are still intact?*

- *If a negative outcome happens, do I have coping strategies and sources of support to help me get through it?*

- *Can I frame the stressful situation in a more positive way?*

- *Are there any positive outcomes that could happen instead of the negative one I'm expecting?*

- *Is there a way to see myself and my actions or abilities in a more positive light?*

- *Is there anything meaningful or helpful I can take from the situation?*

Overthinking things and second-guessing yourself:

- *Am I focusing on what could go wrong, rather than what could go right?*

- *Am I looking for the perfect solution, rather than the best choice given the current circumstances?*

- *Am I willing to accept some reasonable degree of risk and discomfort in order to move forward?*

Unhelpful comparisons:

- *Are other people really doing that much better than I am?*

- *Did they start out with advantages or opportunities that I didn't have?*

- *Am I comparing my insides to other people's outsides? For example, am I comparing how I feel to how other people seem to be doing?*

- *Do I really know what their lives are like?*

- *Am I giving myself enough credit for what I've accomplished or the hard work I've put in?*

Judging mind:

- *Are my judging thoughts helpful, or are they harmful? If they're harmful, can I direct my attention away from them?*

- *Is there a more compassionate and understanding way to view the situation?*

(Remember that your judging thoughts are just thoughts, and you don't have to listen to them. They're not facts, just opinions. Use the mindfulness techniques in this book to imagine your judging thoughts floating by like clouds in the sky.)

Final Thoughts

In this chapter, you learned how your prefrontal cortex and amygdala communicate with each other to exacerbate or calm down your stress reaction. You also learned how secure attachment experiences in childhood or adulthood can create a more flexible, integrated brain response to stress, like mental clay rather than mental sand or cement. Cognitive flexibility is a mental capacity that helps you process conflicting information or look at a situation from multiple perspectives. It helps you take a new tack when the old one isn't working. You learned how worry and rumination can increase your stress response and how to stop catastrophizing and be more realistic in your predictions. You also learned about various thinking traps and how to overcome them.

CHAPTER 8

Bringing in the Positive

As you learned in the previous chapters, stress affects the way you think about your problems. Feeling stressed biases your brain to think in terms of avoiding threat and loss, rather than what you can gain or learn from the situation. It can also give you tunnel vision as your brain homes in on the threat. In this chapter, you'll learn how stress can cause a scarcity mind-set and how to overcome it. You'll also learn to generate positivity when you're under stress, using your prefrontal cortex to tell your amygdala that the situation is safe and it's okay to switch off "fight, flight, or freeze" mode.

Overcoming Hypervigilance

When you feel anxious or stressed, your attention narrows to focus on the threatening situation or dreaded outcome so that you can figure out how to prevent it or minimize your pain and suffering. In evolutionary terms, our ancestors were more likely to survive and not be eaten by lions if they were vigilant for signs of lions. Over hundreds of thousands of years, this narrow focus on the source of threat got wired into our brains as a reaction to stress. The problem is that the stressors you're likely to face today are much more complex and drawn out than the ones your ancestors faced. You're more likely to be dealing with unpaid bills, loneliness, rejection, unemployment, and other situations that don't get resolved right away.

As you learned in chapter 1, constant worry and vigilance can turn an acute stressor into a chronic stressor. Your brain and body don't get a chance to rest or recover, so you're likely to get worn out.

Sue's experiences illustrate how hypervigilance can get in the way of coping with a stressful situation.

Sue was going through a stressful time in her relationship. She and her boyfriend were fighting a lot. She became obsessed with the idea that her boyfriend was cheating on her. She started texting him ten times a day to check on where he was, snooping through his things, and reading his e-mails. She kept starting fights and accusing him of not loving her. She couldn't focus on her job and started making mistakes and getting into trouble with her boss. She stopped seeing her friends and calling her family members, and they began getting annoyed with her. Eventually, her boyfriend got fed up and said he wanted a break from the relationship.

Sue's constant focus on the threat of her boyfriend cheating (which wasn't true, by the way) didn't have the intended effect: it didn't prevent the relationship from ending. It actually may have hastened the relationship's demise. It also made her more insecure and took her away from friends, family members, and work. Her constant focus on her boyfriend's potential cheating stopped her from enjoying the positive aspects of the relationship or building a more loving and affectionate bond.

Is your stress making you hypervigilant to threat or rejection? Are you waiting for the other shoe to drop, feeling as if you can't let up even for a minute? Remind yourself that your brain was designed to alternate working with resting. It wasn't designed to remain hyped up in "fight, flight, or freeze" mode over long periods. You need to find ways to distract yourself and resist the urge to try to control everything. Here are three coping skills that can help.

Letting it be. How might it be for you to let the situation be as it is, without having to do something about it or monitor it all the time? When your amygdala sends your body into "fight, flight, or freeze" mode, you experience an urge to act right away, even if that's not the best thing to do. Take a few deep breaths and slow things down. If trying to control the situation isn't productive, take a step back and just let it unfold. Try to believe that you can deal with whatever happens when and if you need to. Or find a trusted friend or loved one to talk to so that you satisfy your urge to act (in this case, speak) without doing any damage by acting impulsively.

Finding distractions. Instead of monitoring the stressor all the time, find something else to focus on. It might be a fun activity, a challenging task such as a word game, or a hobby such as crafting. You might focus on a news story, follow a TV series, read a book, or watch sports. You might organize your closets. You might interact with your pet, focus on your kids, or think about something funny or sexy.

Fighting your impulses. This skill involves deliberately doing something other than what your amygdala's "fight, flight, or freeze" response tells you to do. It involves using your prefrontal cortex to come up with a different intention and action. If your brain is telling you to constantly monitor your boyfriend's Facebook page, write in your diary instead. If you're tempted to drunk-text your girlfriend when you haven't heard back from her, go home and sleep it off instead. In this way, you're leading with your prefrontal cortex rather than your amygdala, and you're fighting the urge to act destructively in response to stress. This can help you protect your relationships and your health.

In this section, you learned about the costs of hypervigilance and how to use your prefrontal cortex to calm down your amygdala. In the next section, you'll learn about another unhelpful mind-set created by stress.

Overcoming a Scarcity Mind-Set

Many stressful situations involve a feeling of scarcity. You may worry that you don't have enough time, money, companionship, security, and so on, and you may worry that you'll never have enough. Feeling deprived of important resources—love, food, money, and time—can lead to anxiety or anger. You may begin to obsess about the thing you've been deprived of. Or you may feel a need to constantly operate in emergency mode—for example, by pinching pennies unnecessarily, or by scheduling every second of your day and not giving yourself a chance to rest.

In his book (with Eldar Shafir) aptly titled *Scarcity: The New Science of Having Less and How it Defines Our Lives* (2013), Harvard economics professor Sendhil Mullainathan describes how time scarcity and the stress of having to be constantly "on the go" affected his behavior. He started making poor decisions about how to use his time. Not only did he double-book his time and overcommit, but he regularly allowed his car registration to expire and then had to waste time avoiding traffic cops.

A scarcity mind-set narrows our time frame, causing us to make impulsive decisions that increase our difficulties in the long term. Dealing with the stress of scarcity and limited resources increases the problems and barriers you have to deal with, resulting in mental fatigue and cognitive overload. Your prefrontal cortex doesn't operate at its best and lets your fear-driven amygdala drive your decisions. The amygdala will always favor getting rid of short-term stress, rather than creating solutions for the long term. That's why when we're stressed we drink more, neglect our physical and mental health, neglect our needs for intimacy and companionship, or fail to keep our commitments to loved ones. We might put off paying a credit card bill, make only the minimum payment, or even not open the bill, hoping it'll somehow disappear.

Studies show that the stress of being financially strapped, being lonely, or being deprived of food results in an unhealthy obsession with the things you don't have (Kalm and Semba 2005; Shah, Mullainathan, and Shafir 2012; Zawadzki, Graham, and Gerin 2013). Stress and anxiety associated with scarcity also interfere with motivation and willpower, making you more vulnerable to temptation. Perceiving financial scarcity, you may not invest sufficiently to grow your business. Perceiving time scarcity may cause you to neglect your health or not to take downtime, leading to fatigue and burnout. Perceiving a scarcity of love, you may stay in an unhealthy relationship too long.

The stress of scarcity and resultant impaired motivation can also lead to avoidance of actions or situations that could potentially solve the problem or protect you from further damage. Lonely people see themselves and others more negatively and may counterproductively avoid joining group gatherings and activities for fear of rejection. According to the 2015 "Stress in America" survey, 32 percent of Americans say that lack of money prevents them from living a healthy lifestyle, and one in five Americans say they have considered skipping or skipped going to the doctor because of financial stress (American Psychological Association 2015). These decisions can allay short term financial anxiety but lead to long-term health damage.

To combat a scarcity mind-set under stress, you need to take a step back and deliberately think about the big picture and the long-term consequences of your actions. Know that your amygdala will overemphasize the benefit of short-term relief and make you feel you have to resolve a problem right now or that it's dangerous to venture out of your routine and try a new approach. Even when the best way of dealing with a stressor is to change your situation or routine, your brain will naturally resist change and react with "fight, flight, or freeze." That's because for our ancestors, uncertainty and change meant that danger might be lurking. But change and uncertainty don't have the same meanings today. In fact, they're parts of life that we have to get used to in a fast-moving world. To overcome a scarcity mind-set, you need to let your prefrontal cortex and higher thinking centers, rather than your fear-based amygdala, make the decisions.

You need to avoid impulsive actions in favor of well-reasoned ones. Here are some strategies you can use.

Focus on what you have, not what you lack. To create a sense of abundance, focus on all the good things that you already have in your life: love, achievement, family, spirituality, and so on. Most of the time, the stressor is just a small piece of your life.

Clarify your priorities. It's easier to make good decisions under stress when you're clear about what's most important to you. Decide in advance what that is. For example, is it family, security, time freedom, meaningful work, a sense of community, or living a balanced life? If that's your number one priority, what's number two, number three, and so on? Then make decisions about how you spend your time, money, and energy that align with these priorities. It's easier to say no and stop overcommitting when you know where you're headed.

Prepare a strategy in advance. Put measures and routines into place that will help you avoid making impulsive decisions when you feel stressed. Make a list when you go to the supermarket, put appointment reminders in your phone, and schedule regular deposits to your savings account. Don't take your credit card to the mall—take a frugal friend instead. Erase the phone numbers of unavailable love interests (such as married exes) so that you won't call them when you feel weakened by stress.

Take reasonable risks. When you're stressed and resources are scarce, you may not want to take a risk because you have more to lose. Yet often we can't find creative solutions to problems without taking on some degree of risk. Business leaders face this all the time. Companies may get stuck in a rut and fail to innovate when the corporate culture is too opposed to risk. So be willing to try a new approach, to invest your resources, or to hold out for a while if your logic tells you this is the strategy most likely to lead to a positive outcome.

Adopt a long-term perspective. Stress biases us toward alleviating immediate anxiety. You may be focused on immediate deadlines but neglect to deal with issues that are more important in the long term. If you service customers but don't invest in growing your business, you may lose out down the road. You may put all your energy into work and neglect your kids' emotional needs, then face problems when they become teenagers. So think about what's likely to happen one, five, or ten years down the road, and work on finding a solution that reduces stress in the long term.

Build supportive relationships. Under stress, when resources seem scarce, we get competitive with others because we think that more for somebody else means less for us. In fact, the opposite can be true: If you help other people grow their business, they may be more likely to refer extra business to you. Or if you drive carpool when somebody can't make it, you'll have more help when you need it later on. Research shows that social support is one of the strongest buffers against the negative effects of stress on mental and physical health (Cohen and Wills 1985; Rosengren et al. 1993).

Creating Positive States of Mind

Research on "positive psychology" (Fredrickson 2004) suggests that creating or focusing on positive emotions can have three important benefits. These benefits could potentially help us deal better with stress. First, positive emotions help us *recover physiologically* from stress. Second, they encourage us to *engage*—to explore, be curious, and take reasonable risks, rather than fleeing, fighting, or freezing. This can lead us to new information and resources that may help us deal with the stressor. Third, positive emotions can help us *think more broadly* about our stressors, which increases our chances of finding a novel and creative solution. We'll discuss each of these functions in more detail below.

Positive emotions can help your body recover physiologically from stress. In one study (Frederickson et al. 2000), researchers induced stress by telling all the participants (in this case, college students) they would have to give a speech under time pressure, for which they'd be videotaped and evaluated. This led to anxiety and increases in heart rate and blood pressure. The participants then watched one of four films: one designed to provoke amusement, one designed to provoke contentment, one designed to have a neutral effect, or one designed to create sadness. Results showed that participants who watched one of the first two films, intended to provoke positive emotion, had faster cardiovascular recovery (heart rate and blood pressure returned to pre-stress levels) than the others. Creating positive emotions is thus proven to quicken the body's recovery from physiological stress.

The second way that positive emotions that can help us cope with stress is through engagement. Emotion theorists believe that the function of positive emotions is to motivate us to engage actively with our environment, rather than retreating or avoiding. Ways to avoid feeling the anxiety and negative feelings associated with stress include shopping excessively, drinking too much alcohol, overeating, not venturing out of your home, spacing out, sleeping too much, playing video games, and watching TV for hours. These actions can create temporary positive emotions, but at a cost to your health and well-being. Avoidance and procrastination waste energy that you could use to cope actively with the stressor. Later, they make you feel bad about yourself and anxious about the things you didn't get done. If you can learn to feel happier or more positively engaged, then you may be able to cope more actively with stress.

Positive emotions and mental states may make people more resilient to stress, like sturdy tree branches that bend but don't break when battered by a storm. Studies show that more resilient people cope with stress by using humor, doing relaxing activities, and thinking optimistically (for a review, see Masten and Reed 2002). These coping strategies can create positive emotions, such as amusement, interest, contentment, and hope. Resilient people also know how to create positive emotions in family members, friends, and coworkers, which likely earns them more support and empathy when they're under stress. In one study (Tugade and Frederickson 2004), people who scored as more resilient on a questionnaire reported more positive emotions and demonstrated faster cardiovascular recovery from a stressful speech task than less resilient individuals. Statistical analyses showed that the positive emotions created the faster recovery, at least in part. Resilient people may be particularly skillful at using positive emotions to recover from stress.

A third function of positive emotions is to broaden the way we think about problems, which helps us reframe stressful situations more positively or discover creative solutions. Have you ever taken a walk to relax when stuck on a work problem and had a new insight or creative idea when you returned? The state of relaxation you experienced during walking may have opened up your thinking so that you could approach the problem in new ways. That's why it's essential to take a break from your stress and do things you enjoy or be with people you love. The resultant positive states will not only lift you up but also potentially help you find better ways of dealing with your stressors.

Positive emotions also create broad-minded thinking. In one study (Fredrickson and Joiner 2002), researchers measured broad-minded thinking and positive emotions using a questionnaire with items such as "Think of different ways to deal with the problem" and "Try to step back from the situation and be more objective." Participants rated their likelihood of using each strategy to cope with a stressor, and higher scores indicated more broad-minded thinking. Results showed that people who reported more positive emotions were more likely to use broad-minded thinking to deal with problems in the following weeks. Broad-minded thinking, in turn, created even more positive emotions over time. In other words, experiencing positive emotions when under stress can create an upward spiral of effective coping.

Positive emotions may help your prefrontal cortex to do its job in calming down automatic reactivity to stress so that you can focus, integrate different information, and come up with a plan for moving forward. A study of individuals dealing with bereavement showed just this effect. Research participants who reported experiencing some positive emotions despite dealing with bereavement were more likely to develop long-term plans and goals. Both positive emotions and plans and goals, in turn, predicted better mental health twelve months later (Stein et al. 1997).

How can you use these research findings on positive emotions and states of mind to better cope with the stressors you're facing? One way is to build in a "resilience plan" in which you proactively engage in activities that create positive emotions, then deliberately use these positive moods to fuel your thinking about your stressor.

PRACTICE: Creating Positive Moods

The following list shows you what types of activities create different types of positive moods, so that you can choose the ones that will work best for you.

The list isn't exhaustive, and it's okay to substitute other activities that you prefer. Pick two to four activities that might work for you, and then make a plan to fit these into your schedule on a regular basis. Soon after you finish the activity, schedule twenty to thirty minutes to sit and think about how to deal with your stressor. Notice what creative solutions come to mind.

- **Play and creative activities** can create *joy* and help you *push the limits of your mind and problem-solve creatively*.

- **Exploring and trying new things** can create *interest* and help you *integrate new information and expand your horizons*.

- **Enjoying nature or beauty, practicing gratitude, or recalling positive memories** can create *contentment* and help you *have a positive focus and find a new perspective.*

- **Spending time with loved ones** can create *love* and help you *feel energized, inspired, or safe.*

- **Sports or entertainment** can create *relaxation* and help you *slow down and find a new perspective.*

- **Challenging tasks** can create *engagement* and help you *have confidence, be focused, and feel a sense of flow.*

- **Humor** (such as jokes and funny shows) can create *amusement* and help you *find a new perspective, get some distance from your problems, and attain objectivity.*

In the next section, you'll learn to use gratitude to cope with your stress. Gratitude is one of the most well-researched positive states.

Using Gratitude to Gain a New Perspective

Gratitude is a positive state of mind in which you deliberately focus on the good things in your life and feel appreciative. As motivational author Melody Beattie said: "Gratitude unlocks the fullness of life. It turns what we have into enough, and more. It turns denial into acceptance, chaos to order, confusion to clarity" (Beattie 1990, 218). Practicing gratitude can change your perspective on your stressor from one of lack and scarcity to a sense of acceptance, openness, and contentment.

Practicing gratitude offers many potential benefits when you're dealing with stress. It can create the broad-minded thinking that helps you view your life and problems from a more optimistic perspective. It counteracts the tendency to overvalue and obsess about the things that are threatened by the stressor. It can also help you overcome a sense of failure or defeat. Gratitude also helps you protect your relationships from the effects of stress. You're less likely to take your stress out on loved ones when you think about what they mean to you and how they've helped you. Gratitude helps you realize that you have a choice about what to focus your attention on and you don't have to let the stressor take all the joy out of your life. Finally, gratitude can help improve your motivation to cope in healthy ways and to persist when things get difficult. For example, when you feel more content and nourished, you'll be less likely to think that you "need" that extra glass of wine.

One well-known research study (Emmons and McCullough 2003) of over 200 undergraduates examined the benefits of writing gratitude diaries. Students were divided into three groups and instructed to write a weekly diary focusing on one of three topics: gratitude (blessings), hassles and annoyances, or neutral events. At the end of the ten weeks, those who wrote about things they were grateful for reported feeling more positive about their lives as a whole, feeling more optimistic about the upcoming week, having fewer physical complaints (such as a cough or headache), and spending more time exercising. Practicing gratitude can help you feel better about your life. It has a kind of grounding effect that gives your prefrontal cortex more power to rein in the wayward amygdala.

Gratitude helps you be more optimistic—a quality that boosts the immune system, according to research. In one study (Segerstrom et al. 1998), researchers measured the immune functioning of first-year students undergoing the stress of adjusting to law school. They found that, by midterm, students who were classified as more optimistic maintained higher numbers of cells that protect the immune system, compared with their more pessimistic peers. When we're able to look on the bright side, it's easier to maintain the hope and balanced perspective that keeps us going for the long haul.

Given its many benefits, gratitude seems like an important tool for managing stress.

PRACTICE: Writing a Gratitude Diary

On your computer or in a special notebook, begin a diary. Decide how frequently you'll write in this diary (in the research studies, participants wrote either once per day or once per week, but daily writing had more positive effects on mood), then set aside a regular time and place to do it. In the evening is best, so that you can reflect on what you experienced that day (if you're writing daily).

Each time you write, reflect on what happened that day (or that week) and write down as many as five things—large or small—that you feel grateful for. These might be the people you love, your pet, the activities that give your life meaning, people who help you, the abundance of nature, the things that nourish you, or anything else that you choose to write about. Explain, in just one sentence if you like, what each thing adds to your life.

Final Thoughts

In this chapter, you learned how stress and anxiety create hypervigilance. You also learned that stress can create a scarcity mind-set that favors short-term stress relief over long-term health and happiness. Strategies for combating this mind-set include prioritizing and preparing in advance. In the last part of the chapter, you learned how creating positive emotions and positive states of mind can undo the physiological effects of your "fight, flight, or freeze" response, motivate you to cope actively with your stressor, and broaden the way you think about the stressful situation. Finally, you learned how to keep a gratitude diary.

CHAPTER 9

Finding the Right Mind-Set

In this chapter, you'll learn that managing your stress is all about having the right attitude. Your mind-set can determine whether you get overwhelmed by the stressor or turn it into a learning or growth opportunity. This doesn't mean that stress doesn't feel stressful or affect your health and happiness if not managed properly. Rather, it means you can lessen the negative impacts and even create positive outcomes of stress by changing your attitude toward stress. In this chapter, you'll learn about different mind-sets that are part of a stress-proof brain. A *"stress-is-beneficial"* mind-set can help you transform your stress into a growth opportunity and even find benefit in it. Finally, you can learn to be mentally tough and hardy under stress, using *grit* to persevere and keep your eye on the long-term goal.

The "Stress-Is-Beneficial" Mind-Set

How you think about your stress is important. Your prefrontal cortex has the ability to ramp up your amygdala with panicky, negative thoughts or calm it down with calming and optimistic thoughts. In this section, you'll learn how seeing your stress as potentially beneficial can help you cope more effectively.

Whether you think about stress as beneficial or harmful can affect the way you approach the stressor and its ultimate outcome. You can believe that stress will sap your energy and damage your health, or you can believe that stress presents a growth and learning opportunity. If you think *Stress is harmful,* your primary focus will be to try to avoid or minimize feelings of stress. However, if you think *Stress can be beneficial,* you'll be more motivated to face the stressor actively and use the situation to your best advantage or to work on accepting stressors you can't change. For example, if you've just been promoted, rather than focusing on avoiding feeling stressed, you can focus on the opportunity for leadership and learning new skills, to help you perform at your highest potential.

Sometimes you can't change the types of stressors you have to face, so you need to accept they're there and make the best of them. Remember (from chapter 1) the research by Elissa Epel and her colleagues that showed damaging effects of stress on telomeres, an indicator of cellular health and aging, in mothers caring for children with disabilities? Mothers who didn't perceive their caregiving as highly stressful—who likely viewed their caretaking role as meaningful and important, rather than as a burden—were protected from these negative effects.

Stanford psychologist Kelly McGonigal (2015) advises that we focus on embracing stress, rather than trying to reduce it. She suggests three ways to protect yourself from the harmful effects of stress:

- Focus on the positive aspects of your body's stress response, such as the extra energy and motivation it gives you.

- View yourself as somebody who can successfully cope with stress by adapting and growing with each new experience.

- View stress as inevitable and universal; don't take it personally.

If you see stressful events as meaningful or as manageable personal challenges, you'll feel pride and excitement. Although your body may still go into "fight, flight, or freeze" mode, with the same racing heart and sweaty palms, this may feel invigorating rather than overwhelming, like riding a roller coaster or skydiving! And when it's done, you'll feel like a better person for having done the difficult task. If you can do this, you can do something even more difficult the next time. You may start to see yourself as resilient, capable, or even brave.

A recent study (Brooks 2014) showed that interpreting your feelings of anxiety as excitement may actually help your mood and performance more than trying to calm down. Participants preparing to give a speech who followed instructions to interpret their body's stress-related physiological arousal as excitement felt more excited about the task and performed better than those who were instructed to try to calm their stress reactions. When you adopt a mind-set that focuses on the positive outcomes of feeling stressed, stressful feelings will become less of a barrier. On the other hand, if you see stress as harmful, you may develop "fear of fear," in which you interpret feelings of anxiety and stress themselves as threats and signs of failure. You may become stressed about being stressed, leading to a vicious cycle. Feeling too much stress and anxiety can get in your way, but feeling a moderate level of physiological stress and anxiety can actually enhance your performance. You need just enough stress to get your brain chemicals ramped up to put lots of fuel into your tank but not so much that you feel overwhelmed and can't think straight.

Your attitude toward stress is important, because it can influence how you respond to stress. Viewing stress as harmful may lead you to cope in unhealthy ways. You may drink too much, procrastinate to avoid feelings of stress, or ruminate about harmful consequences of stress. These strategies can get in the way of coping proactively with your stressor.

Seeing stress as beneficial can help you accept feelings of stress and use the boost of energy they provide to work hard and give it all you've got. If you focus only on avoiding stress, you won't stretch yourself and you won't achieve at your highest potential. Imagine that you're lonely. If you sit at home, you'll reduce your stress in the short term, but at a cost to your vitality and self-esteem. But if you challenge yourself to go out to the library, coffee shop, dog park, or gym, or do volunteer work, you'll feel like more of a participant in the world, rather than an observer. And you're likely to meet people or find opportunities that improve your mood and self-esteem. Indeed, a study of employees at a financial institution showed that adopting the "stress-is-beneficial" mind-set was associated with greater life satisfaction and fewer psychological symptoms over time (Crum, Salovey, and Achor 2013).

Thinking that stress is harmful creates avoidance that interferes with the opportunity to learn new skills. In one of the studies reported in Crum, Salovey, and Achor's (2013) article, participants given a speech task who had a "stress is beneficial" mind-set were more likely to want feedback that could improve their speaking skills. Those who considered stress to be harmful reduced their exposure to stress by choosing not to get feedback, which inhibited their learning and personal growth.

The good news is that a "stress is beneficial" mind-set can be taught. In another study reported in Crum, Salovey, and Achor (2013), more than three hundred managers at an international financial institution (UBS) were shown one of two 3-minute videos: either a video about the "harmful" effects of stress on health and performance or a video about the "beneficial" effects of stress on health and performance. Not only did those in the "stress-is-beneficial" group display a more positive attitude toward their stress, but they had better mental health and performed better at work in the following weeks.

Now that you know about the importance of your mind-set toward stress, the next section will help you find your "stress-is-beneficial" mind-set by explaining the actual benefits of stress. Afterward is a practice that will help you change your stress mind-set to one of benefit.

The Benefits of Stress

Although stress can be harmful, it can also lead to resilience. In studies, when people (or rats) are exposed to a mild or moderate stressor that they're able to master, they'll cope better with a larger stressor later on, just as a vaccine immunizes us against a disease. If you've never had to deal with any significant changes or obstacles, you may feel less confident and give up more easily when you face a challenging situation late in life. A review of studies on resilience in humans concluded that "resistance...may derive from controlled exposure to risk (rather than its avoidance)" (Rutter 2006).

Exposure to stressful events can help protect you from later stress. In one study, children with moderate levels of early life stressors (compared to those with either lower or higher levels) showed smaller physiological responses to a stressor (Gunnar et al. 2009). A review article on this topic concluded that "a history of *some* lifetime adversity predicts better outcomes than not only a history of *high* adversity but also a history of *no* adversity. This has important implications for understanding resilience, suggesting that adversity can have benefits" (Seery 2011, 390; emphasis in original).

Parents who want to raise resilient kids need to know that kids need opportunities to cope with some frustration and difficulty in life. That's why being a "helicopter parent" actually does your kids a disservice—because it doesn't help them learn to deal with stress. Richard Dienstbier's (1989) theory of mental toughness suggests that experiencing some manageable stresses, with recovery in between, can make us more mentally and physically tough and less reactive to future stress. We learn to view stressors as more manageable and to use better coping strategies.

Even severe stressors can lead to benefits in three life areas: (1) self-image, (2) relationships, and (3) personal development and prioritizing. In one study of people who had suffered the loss of a loved one, 73 percent of participants reported finding at least some positive meaning in the loss six months afterward (Davis, Nolen-Hoeksema, and Larson 1998). Experiencing stressors makes you more likely to rely on support from family members and friends, strengthening your connections to them. A stressful life event can also be a wake-up call, stimulating you to change your life's direction or rearrange your priorities.

Stressors can change your worldview in a number of ways. You may focus less on material things and more on relationships or spirituality. You may become more responsible and give up addictive behaviors. You may begin to see your time as more valuable and spend it more wisely. You may find meaning in the stressor by educating others about it or connecting with people who've experienced similar things. You may even forge a new identity—by making a different career choice, volunteering, or becoming involved in advocacy.

Finding benefits or positive meaning in your stressor may help protect your health. In one study of men who had recently had their first heart attack (Affleck et al. 1987), over half of the men reported benefits of the experience. These included adopting a healthier lifestyle, living a more enjoyable life, and changes in priorities, values, and ways of seeing the world. Those who perceived benefits were less likely to have a second heart attack and more likely to be alive eight years later!

A study of early-stage breast-cancer patients (Stanton et al. 2002) also showed that finding benefits in your stressor can help protect your health. In this study, participants were given a writing exercise. Some of the participants were instructed to write down positive thoughts and feelings relating to their cancer experience. Others were instructed to write down their deepest thoughts and feelings about breast cancer. Participants in both of these groups had fewer doctor visits for cancer-related problems in the three months following the study than those in the control group, who were instructed to write down the facts of their breast cancer experience without mentioning emotions. In other words, finding benefits in the stress of cancer or deliberately expressing deeply held feelings about it led to improved health over time.

Even if you don't have a health-related stressor, such as cancer or a high risk of heart attack, seeing some benefit in your stressor will likely reduce its negative effects. If you're facing a financial problem, this may be an opportunity to change your relationship with money or change your priorities. If you feel stressed by balancing your job with your home life, this may be an opportunity for you to set boundaries. If you're stressed by a leadership role at work, this could be an opportunity for you to grow your skills and make a difference. If you're stressed by parenting responsibilities, you could try to see these responsibilities as meaningful and important. The important thing is that you see the stressor as enhancing your life in some way, as meaningful, or as a learning opportunity.

PRACTICE: **Viewing Your Stressor as Having Some Benefits**

Think about a specific stressor you're facing, and, in a journal or on a separate piece of paper, write your answers to the following questions:

Does this stressor provide any opportunities to stretch yourself and learn new skills—for example, work skills, assertiveness skills, communication skills, time management, or self-control? Explain.

Does this stressor have the potential to make you a stronger, wiser, or better person? Describe how this could come about.

Does this stressor provide the opportunity to deepen your relationship(s) in some way, such as by turning to others for help; helping others; working together; becoming a better leader, partner, or parent; or becoming more kind and empathic? Explain.

How might you use this stressor as an opportunity to improve your health and lifestyle or take better care of yourself?

How might this stressor help you clarify or change your priorities in life so that you can be happier and healthier?

Could this stressor help you grow personally or spiritually? Explain.

It may be hard to find benefit in having experienced a trauma, such as sexual abuse or the loss of a child, and you shouldn't feel forced to do so. If your stressor is having seriously negative impacts on you, don't feel as if you have to engage in denial or minimize its importance. It's normal to have negative feelings, as well as positive ones, about stressors. If you're feeling distressed by your stressor, there's no need to blame yourself for not being more positive. Benefit-finding may not be for everyone, but for some people dealing with some kinds of stressors, it can be a useful way of protecting mental and physical health. In the next section, you'll learn about a different mind-set that can help you persevere in the face of stress.

Becoming Gritty

Another type of mind-set that can help you cope with stress is grit. Many types of stressors require working hard over long periods of time, tolerating frustration and failure, and continuing to pursue your goals despite obstacles. You need determination and mental toughness to "stay in it" for the long haul.

The concept of hardiness suggests that a certain set of attitudes can help you be more resilient to stress. Research (Kobasa 1979) suggests that resilient people have three important characteristics—commitment, challenge, and control. Commitment involves having a passion for what you do that allows you to stick with it when things get rough. Challenge involves viewing your stressor as a challenge, rather than a threat (which helps your amygdala calm down and generates positive emotions, such as hope and excitement). Control involves investing your time and energy in changing the things you can control, rather than trying to change the unchangeable. This helps you direct your efforts where they'll pay off the most. Although you can't control what stressors you experience, you can control how you respond to these stressors.

University of Pennsylvania psychology professor Angela Lee Duckworth and her colleagues (2007) introduced the concept of "grit" to capture the qualities of determination, passion, and purpose. Gritty people are those who are driven to succeed, have a passion for what they're doing, and are willing to stick it out when things get difficult. Gritty people know what their priorities are and keep their long-term goals in mind, rather than second-guessing themselves and getting distracted. Grit can help you stay on course despite being stressed. It's measured by a Grit Scale (http://angeladuckworth.com/grit-scale), which contains statements such as "I have overcome setbacks to conquer an important challenge" and "I finish whatever I begin."

Dr. Duckworth's research subjects include students, military cadets, married couples, and corporate salespeople. Her research shows that being gritty (working hard, being driven, and persevering despite difficulties) is a good predictor of eventual success—better than IQ or family income. Grittier students at the University of Pennsylvania achieved higher GPAs despite lower scores on standardized college entry tests. Grittier cadets at West Point were less likely to drop out of the grueling training program, and grittier salespeople were more likely to make their quotas and keep their jobs (Eskreis-Winkler et al. 2014; Duckworth 2016).

Being gritty means being willing to tolerate some discomfort in order to reach a personally important goal. It means making a conscious decision to tolerate some stress, rather than giving up. When you're gritty, your passion for the goal keeps you motivated and lifts your spirits. Gritty people are better able to see failure as a learning opportunity, rather than being discouraged by it. They spend more time practicing and improving their skills so that they can attain eventual success.

A gritty mind-set is an important part of a stress-proof brain. Grit involves using your prefrontal cortex to calm your amygdala, controlling the impulse to run away from a stressful situation (flight) or be overwhelmed (freeze). It involves deliberately changing your perspective from the short-term stressor to the long-term view. Some stressors are worth putting up with. Working hard to "pay your dues" at work and making the extra effort to show leadership can lead to faster promotion later on. Sticking it out through a difficult stage of a marriage (such as when a new baby is born or when the oldest kids become teenagers) can lead to long-term relationship improvement and happiness.

A gritty mind-set helps you act strategically and preserve your energy for the long haul. Grit is about stamina and having realistic expectations. It's about seeing failure as an inevitable part of life, rather than a disaster. Gritty people take responsibility for their contribution to problem situations and seek to learn and improve, rather than seek to avoid stress. They have the vision and confidence that helps them accept and put up with stress in the service of long-term goals. In the next practice, you'll learn to become grittier in dealing with your stressors.

PRACTICE: **Becoming Grittier**

In a journal or on a separate piece of paper, write a one- or two-line summary of your long-term goal(s). For example, "I want to be a successful dentist," "I want to do what I love," "I want to master oil painting," "I want to be part of a community," or "I want to raise confident kids." Then write your answers to the following questions.

- How committed are you to these goals? Why are they so meaningful or personally important to you?

- How will successfully coping with or tolerating this stressor move you closer to these goals?

- What types of stress or discomfort are you willing to put up with in order to move closer to your goals (failure, rejection, uncertainty, feeling tired, and so on)?

- What are some things you can do to increase your stamina so that you can better withstand stress? What might help you feel more sturdy, steady, strong, energized, or optimistic?

- Can you reframe the way you think about your stressor, so that it feels more like a learning opportunity and less like a permanent obstacle to attaining your goals? (You may need to reframe the way you think about your goals or define them more broadly.)

Final Thoughts

In this chapter, you learned about mind-sets that can help you tolerate and cope with stress. Seeing your stressor as having some benefits can motivate you to accept what you can't change and to take advantage of opportunities to learn and grow. Experiencing controllable stress can help you learn to handle stress so that you'll cope better the next time. Finally, hardiness and a gritty mind-set involve using your commitment to long-term goals as a motivation to persevere and withstand stress.

CHAPTER 10

Living Healthy in the Face of Stress

Stress can be mentally exhausting, making your amygdala more powerful and difficult to regulate. Stress can cause inflammation, insomnia, and weight gain, and it can lead to excess alcohol use. But a lifestyle that includes enough sleep, healthy eating, and regular exercise can strengthen your brain's ability to manage stress and help protect your mental and physical health. In this chapter, you'll learn some ways to live healthier in the face of stress.

Chronic Stress and Inflammation

The stress hormone cortisol signals your immune system to gear up to fight bacteria or heal injury, as well as to return to baseline when the stressor is over. Acute inflammation is your body's natural, self-protective response to physical or emotional stress. Chronic stress can, however, decrease the effectiveness of cortisol in regulating your immune response and reducing inflammation when the stressor is over. Your tissues may become less sensitive to the signaling function of cortisol, causing inflammation to get out of control. Runaway inflammation can contribute to the development of depression, heart disease, diabetes, or cancer, as well as asthma and allergies. But exercise, healthy eating, and stress management can reduce stress-related inflammation, as you'll see in this chapter.

Chronic Stress and Weight Gain

Have you ever found yourself mindlessly eating a tub of ice cream while you brood about your latest romantic rejection or eating a hamburger and fries in front of your computer as you furiously try to meet a work deadline? Perhaps you're a busy mom, eating cookies in your car as you shuttle the kids back and forth to a slew of activities. Stress that goes on for a long time is a triple whammy for weight—it increases your appetite, makes your body hold on to fat, and interferes with your willpower to implement a healthy lifestyle.

Under stressful conditions, your brain releases a cascade of chemicals, including adrenaline and cortisol. In the short term, adrenaline helps you feel less hungry as your blood flows away from your internal organs and to your large muscles to prepare you to fight or flee. However, once the effects of adrenaline wear off, cortisol hangs around and starts signaling your body to replenish your food supply. Fighting off wild animals, as our ancestors did, used up a lot of energy, so their bodies needed more stores of fat and glucose. Today's humans, who often sit on the couch worrying about how to pay the bills or work long hours at the computer, don't work off much energy at all dealing with stressors! Unfortunately, we're stuck with a neuroendocrine system that didn't get the update, so your brain's going to tell you to reach for that plate of cookies anyway.

As mentioned in chapter 1, stress can also cause your body to hang on to belly fat. In the days when our ancestors were fighting tigers and famine, their bodies adapted by learning to store fat supplies for the long haul. The unfortunate result is that when you're chronically stressed, you're prone to develop an extra layer of "visceral fat" deep in your belly. This excess belly fat is unhealthy and difficult to get rid of. It releases chemicals that trigger inflammation. Excess cortisol also slows down your metabolism, because your body wants to maintain an adequate supply of glucose for the hard mental and physical work of dealing with the threat. This means your body burns calories more slowly, making you even more prone to weight gain.

Stress can also lead to feelings of anxiety. Adrenaline is the reason for the "wired" feeling you get when you're stressed. Although you may burn some extra calories fidgeting or running around cleaning because you can't sit still, anxiety can trigger "emotional eating."

Overeating or eating unhealthy foods in response to stress or as a way to calm down is very common. In the American Psychological Association's 2015 "Stress in America" survey, almost 40 percent of respondents reported dealing with stress in this way. Engaging in sedentary activities to deal with stress is also quite common. About two in five respondents (39 percent) reported watching TV for more than two hours a day to deal with stress, while 40 percent reported going online or surfing the Internet. Being a couch potato increases the temptation to overeat. Surfing the Internet or watching TV can also make you eat more "mindlessly"—without really noticing the taste of the food, how much you've eaten, or when you're feeling full. When you eat mindlessly, you'll likely eat more yet feel less satisfied.

When we're chronically stressed, we crave "comfort foods," such as a bag of potato chips or a tub of ice cream. These foods tend to be easy to eat, highly processed, and high in fat, sugar, or salt. A University of Pennsylvania research study (Teegarden and Bale 2008) showed that mice who were "stressed" by the experimenters chose food pellets with more fat content. In addition, you may associate certain foods from your childhood with calm and comfort. Remember those freshly baked cookies at Grandma's house?

Stress may also lead you to eat less healthily because you lack time and energy. When you're stressed, you're more likely to eat fast food, rather than taking the time and energy to plan and cook a meal. Americans are less likely to cook and eat dinner at home than people from many other countries, and they also work more hours. If you work in an urban area, you may have a long, jammed commute, which both increases your stress and interferes with your willpower because you're hungrier when you get home.

So, to recap: stress can cause overeating, unhealthy eating, a more sedentary lifestyle, a slower metabolism, and more belly fat. But you can compensate for these effects by putting time and energy into a stress-management routine that may include exercise or meditation. And with a bit of preparation, you can begin to eat better. You'll learn about these strategies later in this chapter.

Stress and Sleep Disturbance

According to the APA's 2015 "Stress in America" survey, nearly half of American adults (46 percent) lie awake at night as a result of stress. Stress upsets the balance between your sympathetic nervous system's "fight, flight, or freeze" response and your parasympathetic nervous system's signals to return your body to baseline so that you can "rest and digest." You become hyperaroused and can't switch off your stress response at the end of the day.

Stress can affect your ability to fall asleep and stay asleep. Insomnia can create further stress by interfering with your brain's ability to focus and regulate your mood. Even if you don't have insomnia, stress can interfere with the quality of your sleep, making it less restful and refreshing. Almost half of American adults (46 percent) report sleeping only fairly or poorly when they're stressed, according to the APA's 2015 Stress in America survey.

You may also lose sleep because of staying up all night to cram for exams or working until the early hours. Stress decreases blood sugar, which leads to fatigue during the day. If you drink coffee or caffeinated soft drinks to stay awake, or if you drink alcohol to feel better, your sleep cycle will be further disrupted. Lack of sleep may disrupt the functioning of ghrelin and leptin—chemicals that control appetite. We crave carbs when we're tired or grumpy from lack of sleep. Finally, not getting those precious z's erodes your willpower and ability to resist temptation, adding to the negative effects of cortisol on your prefrontal cortex.

Stress and Alcohol Use

A research study (Keyes et al. 2012) found that both men and women who reported higher levels of stressful life events drank more alcohol. But men turned to alcohol as a means of dealing with stress more often than women did. For example, among those who reported experiencing at least six stressful life events, the percentage of men who engaged in binge drinking was about 1.5 times that of women, and alcohol-use disorders among men were 2.5 times higher than among women. Men may have fewer natural outlets for emotional expression than women, making them more likely to drink as a way of reducing their anxiety or allowing themselves to express pent-up feelings caused by stress.

Perhaps an occasional glass of wine can take the edge off your feelings of stress and anxiety. It may make you feel more relaxed and happy, more at ease, and more social, rather than preoccupied with your problems. On the other hand, the more you drink, the higher the dose of alcohol you need to get the relaxing effect. And being drunk may lead to fights with your partner, legal problems, or weight gain. You may not sleep as well at night. The next day, you may have a hangover or feel more depressed and anxious. Drinking to excess is a way of escaping your problems, rather than dealing with them directly. Thus, alcohol is more of a short-term fix than a long-term solution. Becoming intoxicated can also create more stress and wear and tear on your body, because your body has to use extra energy to metabolize the alcohol. And when you're intoxicated, your body releases more cortisol, even though you may initially feel happier.

For women, heavy drinking is defined as having more than three drinks at a time and more than seven drinks a week. For men, it's defined as having more than four drinks at a time and more than fourteen drinks a week. Over the long term, heavy drinking makes your brain and body more reactive to stress. It acts as a chronic stressor on your body, interfering with your normal stress response and reducing your body's ability to return to balance following stress. Therefore, chronic stress combined with heavy drinking is a double whammy for your health and can lead to early aging. It's important that you control your alcohol use and find healthier ways to relax when you're stressed. This means developing new habits, which takes time, effort, and persistence.

Exercising to Manage Your Stress

Chronic stress and unhealthy ways of managing your stress, such as overeating and drinking too much alcohol, can negatively affect your health. In this section, you'll learn how regular exercise can help buffer your brain and body against the effects of chronic stress.

Regular aerobic exercise, such as walking, running, or swimming, can feel exhilarating and help you relax. It can also improve your mood. That's why exercise is sometimes used to treat anxiety disorders and clinical depression. Exercise reduces your levels of adrenaline and cortisol and increases your levels of calming and "feel-good" chemicals such as norepinephrine, serotonin, and dopamine. It also may increase your body's production of endorphins that reduce pain and endocannabinoids thought to produce "runner's high," the sense of calm, well-being, strength, and optimism that you sometimes feel after an aerobic workout. Animal studies (Pagliari and Peyrin 1995) show that exercise stimulates the brain's production of norepinephrine, which improves the communication between other brain chemicals, helping our brains respond more effectively to stress.

Exercise can make you feel stronger and more confident in the face of stress. It helps you build physical strength and endurance and maintain a healthy weight. Exercise also provides a boost of energy that can help you get your work and household tasks done more effectively. The self-discipline that exercise involves can help you be grittier and keep moving toward your goals when life gets stressful.

Aerobic exercise may also help protect your brain from premature aging associated with chronic stress (Puterman et al. 2010). Researchers found that women facing chronic stress who exercised vigorously for an average of around forty-five minutes over a three-day period (similar to national health recommendations) had cells that showed fewer signs of aging compared to stressed women who were inactive. Many of these women were caring for relatives with dementia or Alzheimer's disease. As discussed in chapter 1, telomeres (protective caps at the end of our chromosomes) are worn down and shortened by chronic stress, causing our cells to age quicker. This study showed that regular, vigorous exercise may buffer us at a cellular level against the negative effects of stress. Exercise also helps keep us from ruminating by altering blood flow to those areas in the brain involved in bringing up stressful thoughts again and again.

Both intense workouts and recreational exercise can engage you in a way that distracts you from your stress. Exercise may help get you outdoors to enjoy the sunshine or natural beauty. Many runners and bikers like to exercise close to oceans, rivers, or lakes, or on mountain trails. Team sports, such as soccer, baseball, and basketball, or social sports, such as golf and tennis, can help you find new friendships and have fun. Also, moving your large muscle groups (such as those in your arms and legs) in a repetitive rhythm can help you feel more calm and meditative.

Not only sports and aerobic exercise but also stretching exercises such as yoga and Pilates can help you reduce stress. These types of exercise require a mindful focus on the body so as to maintain stability of the muscles in your spine and abdomen (your "core") while moving your arms, legs, or torso. The movements are smooth, stretching, and flowing, leading to a relaxed body awareness and focused attention. The philosophy of Pilates and yoga is to understand and accept your current capacity and slowly work toward improvement, rather than trying to force it. Such an approach builds self-awareness and acceptance, which you can apply to managing your stress.

Yoga and Pilates also require a focus on your breath, which can help your parasympathetic nervous system put the brakes on your "fight, flight, or freeze" response. The combination of deep breathing and rhythmic stretching movements can lead to deep relaxation and stress relief. In one study exploring the benefits of yoga for women with trauma histories, "women experienced improved connections with and sense of ownership and control over their bodies, emotions, and thoughts, and a greater sense of well-being, calmness, and wholeness in their bodies and minds" (Rhodes 2015, 247). More intensive forms of yoga and Pilates also have an energizing quality, because they improve the flow of oxygen through the body.

Now that you know the benefits of exercise, following are some tips to help you build an exercise habit.

Building an Exercise Habit

Regular exercise is an important part of any stress-management routine. It can help protect you from depression and lessen your health risk due to chronic stress. Yet you may struggle to begin a new exercise routine or exercise regularly when you're stressed. You may feel as if you don't have enough time or that exercise cuts into the small amount of time you have with your partner and kids following a long day at work. You may have good intentions but get distracted by other projects, find it difficult to get up early to exercise, or feel too tired to exercise at the end of a stressful day. Your "fight, flight, or freeze" response may make it harder to stop working or getting errands done in order to take time to care for your health; you may be fearful that you won't finish your work if you take a break. In reality, exercise can give you more energy, focus, and mental clarity to tackle your daily demands and manage stressors.

There are other mental barriers to exercising. When you're already stressed out, exercising may feel like just another chore. You may feel self-conscious about your weight or feel ashamed of how unfit you are and not want to face these feelings. You may be scared of feeling uncomfortable and out of breath. In the morning, you may be suffering from a hangover, or you may feel too hungry to work out. At the end of the day, you may simply prefer to watch TV.

Because of these mental, physical, and emotional barriers to exercising when under stress, it's easy to find excuses not to do it. Good intentions aren't enough. You have to take specific steps to translate these desires into action and make a plan to deal with the inevitable obstacles.

In his best-selling book *The Power of Habit*, business writer Charles Duhigg (2012) describes building a new habit as a three-part process. First you give yourself a *cue* that motivates you to do the behavior—for example, you leave your running shoes next to the breakfast nook so that you're reminded to go for your morning jog. Second is the *routine*, which is the actual behavior, such as running two miles every other day on your regular route. Third is the *reward*, which can be the accomplishment and pride you feel as you take your shower or drink a glass of cold water afterward. You may feel rewarded by looking at your toned abs or noticing your stomach shrinking. You may feel energized and alert after exercising, which is an internal reward. Or you may feel rewarded by getting regular feedback. Wearing a pedometer (or, as is popular nowadays, a fitness tracker on your wrist) to record your daily activity and/or calories burned is one way to achieve this.

Even if you don't feel as if you have time for a formal exercise routine, increasing the number of steps you walk each day can help you get fitter, prevent stress-related weight gain, and relieve stress. Brisk walking is an aerobic activity that gets your heart rate up and oxygen pumping through your body. Some experts recommend walking ten thousand steps (about five miles) a day, but it's not a hard and fast rule. If you have a sedentary lifestyle, you may currently take as few as two thousand steps a day. Going from two thousand to ten thousand is a five-fold increase, so you may want to begin by taking five hundred steps more each day and gradually go up to the level that feels most comfortable for you.

PRACTICE: Developing and Maintaining an
Exercise Habit

Here are a number of tips to help you exercise more or build a regular
exercise routine. Circle the numbers of the ones that you feel will best
fit with your preferences and lifestyle.

1. Build more exercise into your daily routine. For example, take the
    steps instead of the elevator, park farther from the office, bike to
    work, climb the stairs in your house more often, walk your dog for
    ten minutes longer, or walk uphill.

2. Find some specific cues to prompt you to exercise. These might
    include writing "EXERCISE!" on a sticky note that you put next
    to your bed, or it might mean pinning up a magazine photo of a fit
    person exercising.

3. Find an intrinsic (internal) motivator, rather than just an extrin-
    sic (external) one. An example of an intrinsic motivator is a desire
    to have more energy or to manage your stress. An extrinsic moti-
    vator might be your doctor saying you need to exercise, or it might
    be your envy of your neighbor's toned abs. Research shows we're
    more likely to stick with exercise when we're internally motivated—
    doing it for ourselves, rather than somebody else.

4. Find an exercise activity that you naturally enjoy. If you don't
    enjoy team sports or are physically uncoordinated, consider
    running, yoga, hiking, or biking. Think about whether you enjoy
    gentle or vigorous exercise and whether you like variety or doing
    the same routine each day. Some people like the structure of exer-
    cise classes or the social atmosphere of the gym, whereas others
    like the flexibility of exercising alone. If you like the social aspect,
    join a team or find an exercise buddy.

5. Be clear what regular reward(s) you're getting from exercising. Pay attention to how much calmer you feel after a run or workout. Or savor the fun time and distraction from stress. Feel good about still fitting into your old jeans or about having extra energy during the day.

6. Think about your barriers to exercising, and find a plan to address them. If you're unfit, start with a small, manageable goal, such as walking for twenty minutes a day. If you're self-conscious about your weight, buy an outfit that makes you feel more attractive. If you're busy, decide which specific days and times you'll exercise, and write these on your schedule. If you get bored exercising alone, find a class or friend to exercise with. If you're tired or hungry at the end of the day, exercise in the morning or at lunchtime. If joining a gym is too expensive, buy an exercise DVD or exercise outdoors.

7. Write a personal exercise contract stating how much and how often you plan to exercise. You can download the template shown at http://www.newharbinger.com/32660.

Improving Your Sleep

As you saw in the previous section, exercising has many psychological and brain benefits when it comes to managing stress. Exercise can also help you get to sleep more easily and get better sleep. In a national study of 2,600 men and women (Loprinzi and Cardinal 2011), following the national guideline of 150 minutes of moderate to vigorous activity a week reduced daytime sleepiness and provided a 65 percent improvement in sleep quality. But even aside from exercise, getting enough good sleep should be a key ingredient of your stress-management plan.

Lack of sleep affects your prefrontal cortex's ability to manage your stress response and keep your amygdala in check. It also interferes with your willpower, mental function, and ability to resist overeating or drinking too much when you're stressed. Even getting less than six hours of sleep a night can act as a chronic stressor, adding to the other stressors that you face. If you're wondering how much sleep is sufficient, a study of over a million people (Kripke et al. 2002) found that people who slept between six and a half hours and seven and a half hours a night lived the longest. Those who reported sleeping for more than eight hours or less than about four hours a night had a higher risk of dying in the subsequent six years.

If stress is interfering with your sleep, you may be tempted to take a sleeping pill such as Ambien (zolpidem), but this is a short-term fix that doesn't deal with the core problem. When you stop taking sleeping pills, your sleep difficulties will return. In addition, sleeping pills can be addictive and can make you feel groggy or depressed the next day. In the study described above, those who took hypnotics such as Ambien were more likely to die, but we don't know for sure whether the medication caused the higher mortality risk. A better strategy is to use some behavioral tools for helping your brain learn new sleep habits.

A good beginning sleep strategy is to eliminate or reduce the activities or substances that interfere with your sleep. These may differ for each person. A common culprit is caffeine. Caffeine is a stimulant found not only in coffee but in many sodas and energy drinks and even in chocolate. Check the label to see whether what you eat and drink contains caffeine. Caffeine not only keeps you awake but makes you sleep more lightly and makes you wake up to go to the bathroom during the night. It's best to reduce your caffeine intake in general as well as not drink or eat anything with caffeine for at least four hours before bedtime. It's best to wean yourself off caffeine or reduce your intake by tapering—gradually decreasing your daily amount.

Alcohol is another culprit when it comes to disturbed sleep. Although alcohol can make you sleepy and help you get to sleep, you're more likely to sleep poorly and to wake up during the night. Binge drinking can reduce your levels of melatonin—a hormone that controls your body clock and affects your production of other hormones—for up to a week, affecting your ability to sleep. Melatonin is decreased by bright light and increased by darkness. So close the blinds and turn off the light. You'll also sleep better without the glow from your electronics, so cover your alarm clock and cell phone. Some people take melatonin supplements; you may want to consult your doctor to see whether this solution is suitable for you.

When you're chronically stressed, your prefrontal cortex becomes hyperalert. Your mind is abuzz with planning or worrying about what you have to do or mentally reviewing stressful interactions. This can interfere with the ability to fall asleep or stay asleep. A small, unpublished research study (American Academy of Sleep Medicine 2011) investigated the idea that overuse of your brain's higher-level functions might make your brain too hot at night. (Your body clock naturally makes you feel warmer during the day and colder at night, to help you fall asleep more easily.) The study showed that using "cooling caps" with circulating cold water helped people fall asleep and stay asleep. Although these results need to be confirmed by more studies, it may help to lower the thermostat to around 65 degrees or drink a glass of cold water before you go to sleep. Only your head needs to stay cool, so you can tuck the rest of your body under a down comforter or snuggle up to your partner if you feel cold.

You also may have routines that interfere with sleep, such as staying up too late at night watching TV, surfing the web, or playing with apps on your phone. A relaxing bedtime routine that may include taking a warm bath, smelling lavender, listening to classical or other types of soft music, doing some yoga stretches, playing nature sounds, or meditating can help you switch off your hyperaroused brain. Once you're in bed, resist the temptation to watch TV, check your phone, or even read a book that stimulates your brain. Lying in bed awake (especially watching your alarm clock, worrying about lack of sleep) can make your brain associate your bed with being awake. That's why experts recommend that you get up after fifteen minutes of not sleeping and do a quiet activity (such as read a book) in another room before going back to bed.

Stress can create aches and pains that make it more difficult to get to sleep. It can also create muscle tension, sometimes even without your awareness of it. In the following practice, you'll learn a brief form of *progressive muscle relaxation*, a proven technique for producing a relaxation response that can help you sleep. Think of it as a way to engage your parasympathetic ("rest and digest") nervous system to put the brakes on your "fight, flight, or freeze" response. After doing this practice, you may feel a sense of calm and relaxation. It takes time to become skilled at relaxing, so it's best to practice several times a week.

PRACTICE: Progressive Muscle Relaxation

During this practice, you'll be tensing and relaxing almost all the major muscle groups in your body. You'll begin with your feet and systematically move up your body to your head. The goal of this exercise is to help you relax and also to teach you the difference between tension and relaxation. During the day, if you begin to notice tension in your muscles, you can practice tensing and relaxing them. Practice this exercise every night at first. It's fine if you fall asleep while doing it.

Begin to tighten and then relax the following areas of your body, one at a time. When you relax, let the feelings of relaxation flow through your muscles like a wave. Just let yourself slowly release all those feelings of tension. Notice what relaxation feels like and how it's different from tension. Then just enjoy the feelings of relaxation in that area of your body.

1. Your right foot (Curl your toes in and clench your foot; then stretch it out.)

2. Your left foot (Repeat what you did on the right.)

3. Your lower right leg (Tense your calf then let it go.)

4. Your lower left leg (Repeat what you did on the right.)

5. Your upper right leg (Squeeze your thigh muscles; then stretch them out.)

6. Your upper left leg (Repeat what you did on the right.)

7. Your groin area and buttocks (Tighten and pull your buttocks in; then slowly release them.)

8. Your abdomen (Pull your belly in; then release it slowly.)

9. Your lower back (Scrunch up your lower back; then release.)

10. Your ribcage (Squeeze your ribs tightly together; then release.)

11. Your upper back (Squeeze your shoulder blades together; then release.)

12. Your right arm (Tighten your entire arm; then release.)

13. Your left arm (Repeat what you did on the right.)

14. Your right hand (Clench and make a fist; then release.)

15. Your left hand (Repeat what you did on the right.)

16. Your shoulders and neck (Raise your shoulders to your ears and scrunch up your neck; then lower and elongate.)

17. Your face (Scrunch up your face and purse your lips; then release.)

Once you've done this practice several times and are familiar with what tension and relaxation feel like, the next time you do the practice you can stop tensing—just relax each muscle group in turn. You can also shorten the exercise by combining muscle groups (do your legs all at once, do your stomach and torso all at once, your shoulders and arms all at once, and so on). You can also buy a progressive muscle relaxation CD or app that will guide you through a practice similar to this one.

Eating Healthier When You Feel Stressed

As you learned earlier, stress can cause you to overeat for emotional reasons and to crave more fatty, starchy, and sugary foods. In this section, you'll learn coping strategies that can help you eat healthier. It's not about trying to diet or starve yourself or getting freaked out if you put on two or three pounds when under stress. It's more about learning a routine and lifestyle that helps you eat mindfully and using food as a way to take a break from stress and nourish yourself.

Many people have learned to stuff down their feelings of fear, anger, or sadness by eating. If you grew up in a family in which the expression of strong emotions was regarded as unacceptable or a sign of weakness, or if you evaluate negative feelings as "bad" or "dangerous" and try to shut them down, you may often try to suppress your emotions. Unfortunately, emotional suppression isn't an effective strategy, because unprocessed feelings often "rebound" at higher intensity. Not knowing how to deal with these more intense feelings, you may turn to emotional eating.

PRACTICE: Mindful Eating

Here's a mindful eating strategy that can change your relationship with food and make it less likely you'll eat for emotional reasons or impulsively grab junk food when you're stressed. To prepare, cut a fruit (such as a fresh green or red apple or pear) into a few thin, crisp slices.

1. Look at one of the slices of fruit, and notice the sensations and thoughts you have. Perhaps you feel an increase in saliva in your mouth, the anticipation of something fresh and crunchy, or a desire for sweetness or tartness. Notice the color and freshness of the fruit.

   Before you take a bite, think about how the fruit got to your table. If it's an apple, think about it growing on the branch of an apple tree in a sunny field. Then think about the people who grew it, picked it, and transported it to you.

2. Bite into the slice, and then close your eyes. Don't begin chewing yet; just focus on that bite of fruit. Notice its taste, texture, and temperature.

3. Chew the bite slowly, just noticing what it feels like. If your mind wanders off or turns to other thoughts, quietly bring it back to the taste of the fruit and how it makes you feel.

4. As you prepare to swallow, try to follow the food's progress as it travels to the back of your mouth and tongue into your throat. Swallow the food, paying attention to how it feels until you can no longer feel any food-related sensation.

5. Take a deep breath and exhale. Notice any feelings that come up.

   Try to eat the first bite or two of every meal in this way. This will help you be mindful for the rest of the meal. Mindful eating also means not doing anything except eating, so rather than multitasking, put the food on a plate and eat it sitting down at the table. Let your mind register that you're taking a break to eat, and pay attention to your food. Focusing mindfully on the process of eating helps you tune in to your body's intuitive signals so that you're more likely to know when you're full.

The following strategies can also help you fight the tendency to overeat or eat unhealthy foods when you feel stressed.

Eat meals on a regular schedule. Those of us who eat late at night are less likely to have regular meal and snack times and are more prone to eating unhealthy foods. When you eat late at night, you also don't get a chance to work off the calories before bed. Taking healthy snack and meal breaks during the day can create a sense of inner calm and contentment that will make you less likely to eat impulsively when you feel out of balance or emotionally deprived.

Plan your meals. Poor planning can cause you to eat junk food because you don't have the energy to shop for and cook healthy food or because there's no healthy food left in the fridge. I can't overstate how important it is to plan your meals and take the time to buy fresh fruit, proteins, whole grains, and vegetables in order to provide yourself with an appetizing alternative to junk food.

Be aware of your trigger foods. Most of us have foods we particularly crave that trigger us to overeat. Doughnuts and other sugary foods can cause your blood sugar to spike and then crash, leading to more hunger down the road. Don't eat for emotional relief, and when you do eat the unhealthy foods you crave, do so in small portions.

Drink less alcohol. Drinking too much alcohol causes you to put on weight. Alcohol also reduces inhibition, making you more likely to throw caution to the wind and eat unhealthy foods.

Practice healthy stress management. Instead of using food and alcohol to unwind after a stressful day, plan other relaxing activities. Go for a walk or to the movies, meet a friend, take a hot bath, do yoga or meditate, listen to music, or light a scented candle. As you learned earlier in this book, meditating by focusing on your breath can soothe your amygdala and give your prefrontal cortex more ability to calm down your stress response.

Final Thoughts

In this chapter, you learned how stress can create inflammation and make you more prone to unhealthy behaviors, such as overeating, drinking too much alcohol, not sleeping enough, and not finding time for exercise. You learned about the importance and benefits of exercising, eating healthy, and getting enough sleep when you're under stress. You also learned coping tools, including setting a specific exercise goal; using cues, routines, and rewards to strengthen a new habit; choosing an activity you enjoy; setting up your environment to promote sleep; and eating more mindfully.

Conclusion

The ability to successfully manage stress is one of the most important skills that you need for happiness and success in today's rapidly changing world. Sudden, unexpected, or long-lasting stress can affect your mood, health, relationships, and quality of life. Your brain's hardwired response to stress triggers you into states of "fight, flight, or freeze" that can lead to impulsive behavior, constant anxiety and rumination, or helplessness and inability to act. Chronic stress and the effects of cortisol, as well as unhealthy ways of managing stress, can threaten your long-term health. On the other hand, if you deal with stress properly, you can calm your emotions, make wiser choices, feel more in control of your life, and take better care of yourself for the long haul. Stress challenges us to persevere in the face of failure, disappointment, and hardship and creates a powerful impetus for personal and psychological growth.

In this book, you learned how stress works in the brain and the automatic stress response initiated by your amygdala and hypothalamus and coordinated in your body by your sympathetic and parasympathetic nervous systems. You learned how neurotransmitters such as adrenaline and hormones such as cortisol ramp you up to fight or escape from an impending threat. You learned how to use mindfulness, emotional awareness, self-compassion, perceiving control, and other strategies to calm your amygdala's perceptions of threat. You also learned how your prefrontal cortex—the executive center of your brain—can help you rein in your brain's automatic stress response so that you can move forward more thoughtfully and strategically, find creative solutions, persevere, stay healthy, and find the positive and growth-enhancing aspects of your stressful situation. You learned how to break the cycle of rumination and how to reduce perfectionism and self-criticism, which can get in the way of taking effective action.

Having a stress-proof brain means being able to slow things down, ground yourself, and overcome feelings of anxiety and helplessness that may have their roots in past, difficult experiences. It means being the CEO of your own brain, rather than letting your amygdala be in charge. You can learn to reorient your thinking from fear and pessimism to openness, hope, curiosity, and creativity. This change in mind-set can help you stay healthier, be happier, have better relationships, be successful in business, or be a leader in your company or community. You can't avoid your stresses, but you can learn to see them as challenges that help you grow and become the best version of yourself!

Acknowledgments

This book represents the accomplishment of a lifelong dream. It has taken several years to come to fruition. Because my work on this book coincided with building my clinical practice in Mill Valley, California, I've needed to rely extensively on my family for support. I'm deeply grateful to my husband, Brian Hilbush, for actively encouraging me, providing a tremendous amount of ongoing practical support and child care to keep our family life running smoothly, and being my lifelong love and inspiration. I'm also deeply grateful to my daughter, Sydney, for doing without her mom on so many evenings and weekends, for putting up with a mom with too many things on her mind, and for letting my work inspire her.

I deeply appreciate the staff at New Harbinger for believing in me and helping shape my ideas and writing. My writing has improved by leaps and bounds under your tutelage. Acquisitions editor Wendy Millstine helped me sharpen my ideas and guided me through the proposal stage. Editor Jess O'Brien, shepherded me through the process with patience and enthusiasm. A special thanks to copy editor Will DeRooy for skillfully editing the manuscript to make it more succinct and readable and for his positive attitude and attention to detail. Editor Nicola Skidmore helped me make the writing more lively, coherent, and engaging. I would also like to thank art director Amy Shoup for a perfect cover. My gratitude also to project manager Jesse Burson, associate editor Vicraj Gill, marketing and publicity associate Fiona Hannigan, and copywriter Lisa Gunther for their help at various stages of this project. I'd also like to thank my agent, Giles Anderson, for his support and encouragement.

I want to thank Frank Sonnenberg for his generous mentoring at the early stages of writing my proposal; my good friend Eileen Kennedy Moore, for generously sharing her work and experience with me; Susan Whitbourne and Lybi Ma, for providing the opportunity to blog for *Psychology Today*; and my blogging and coaching friends, especially LaRae Quy for sharing my work on social media and being a support system for me. Thanks to Phil Manfield for his expert supervision of my clinical work. I'd also like to thank all the mentors who helped me at different stages of my academic career, especially Sharon Foster, Perry Nicassio, Dick Gevirtz, and Arthur Stone. I'm grateful for the love and generosity of my mother-in-law Barbara Hilbush and that of Audrey Penrose in South Africa. I appreciate the support of the Hilbush and Ligatich families and my good friends in Marin, San Diego, London, Cape Town, and Sydney—you know who you are!

My parents Rheda and Ralph Greenberg, who are with me in spirit, always believed in my potential and supported my work. When I was young, my mother put countless hours into helping me with schoolwork, reading to me, taking me to the library, and giving me a love of writing.

Finally, I want to thank my students and clients for how much they have taught me. My clients continue to inspire me with their courage and resilience.

Resources

Buddha's Brain: The Practical Neuroscience of Happiness, Love, and Wisdom, by R. Hanson (Oakland, CA: New Harbinger Publications, 2009)

Getting Past Your Past: Take Control of Your Life with Self-Help Techniques from EMDR Therapy, by F. Shapiro (New York: Rodale Books, 2012)

Greater Good: The Science of a Meaningful Life (blog) (http://greater good.berkeley.edu)

Grit: The Power of Passion and Perseverance, by A. Duckworth (New York: Scribner, 2016)

Marin Psychologist (my blog) (http://marinpsychologist.blogspot.com)

Kelly McGonigal: How to Make Stress Your Friend (TED talk) (https://www.ted.com/talks/kelly_mcgonigal_how_to_make_stress_your_friend).

Mindsight: The New Science of Personal Transformation, by D. Siegel (New York: Bantam, 2010)

Scarcity: The New Science of Having Less and How It Defines Our Lives, by S. Mullainathan and E. Shafir (New York: Picador, Reprint Edition, 2013)

Self-Compassion: The Proven Power of Being Kind to Yourself, by K. D. Neff (New York: William Morrow, 2011)

Spirit Rock: An Insight Meditation Center (http://www.spiritrock.org)

Stress Management and Coping with Stress/Psych Central (http://psychcentral.com/stress)

Thanks! How the New Science of Gratitude Can Make You Happier, by R. A. Emmons (New York: Mariner Books; Reprint edition, 2008)

The Center for Mindful Self-Compassion (http://www.centerformsc .org)

The Happiness Advantage: The Seven Principles of Positive Psychology That Fuel Success and Performance at Work, by Shawn Achor (New York: Broadway Books, 2010)

The Mindful Self-Express (blog), (https://www.psychologytoday.com /blog/the-mindful-self-express)

The Mindful Path to Self-Compassion: Freeing Yourself from Destructive Thoughts and Emotions, by C. K. Germer (New York: Guilford Press, 2009)

University of California San Diego Center for Mindfulness (https:// health.ucsd.edu/specialties/mindfulness/Pages/default.aspx)

References

Adams, C. E., and M. R. Leary. 2007. "Promoting Self-Compassionate Attitudes Toward Eating Among Restrictive and Guilty Eaters." *Journal of Social and Clinical Psychology* 26: 1120–44.

Affleck, G., H. Tennen, S. Croog, and S. Levine. 1987. "Causal Attribution, Perceived Benefits, and Morbidity Following a Heart Attack." *Journal of Consulting and Clinical Psychology* 55: 29–35.

Altenor, A., E. Kay, and M. Richter. 1977. "The Generality of Learned Helplessness in the Rat." *Learning and Motivation* 8: 54–61.

American Academy of Sleep Medicine. 2011. "Cooling the Brain During Sleep May Be a Natural and Effective Treatment for Insomnia." News release. *ScienceDaily*, 13 June, https://www.sciencedaily.com/releases/2011/06/110613093502.htm.

American Psychological Association. 2015. *Stress in America: Paying with Our Health.* Washington, DC: Author.

Baumeister, R. F., E. Bratslavsky, M. Muraven, and D. M. Tice.1998. "Ego Depletion: Is the Active Self a Limited Resource?" *Journal of Personality and Social Psychology* 74: 1252–65.

Beattie, Melody. 1990. *The Language of Letting Go: Daily Meditations on Codependency.* Center City, MN: Hazelden.

Borkovec, T. D., O. M. Alcaine, and E. Behar. 2004. "Avoidance Theory of Worry and Generalized Anxiety Disorder." In *Generalized Anxiety Disorder: Advances in Research and Practice*, edited by R. Heimberg, C. Turk, and D. Mennin. New York: Guilford Press.

Borkovec, T. D., and S. Hu. 1990. "The Effect of Worry on Cardiovascular Response to Phobic Imagery." *Behaviour Research and Therapy* 28 (1): 69–73.

Borkovec, T. D., E. Robinson, T. Pruzinsky, and J. A. Dupree. 1983. "Preliminary Exploration of Worry: Some Characteristics and Processes." *Behaviour Research and Therapy* 21: 9–16.

Brach, T. 2003. *Radical Acceptance: Embracing Your Life with the Heart of a Buddha*. New York: Bantam.

Bratman, G. N., G. C. Daily, B. J. Levy, and J. J. Gross. 2015. "The Benefits of Nature Experience: Improved Affect and Cognition." *Landscape and Urban Planning* 138: 41–50.

Brooks, A. W. 2014. "Get Excited: Reappraising Pre-Performance Anxiety as Excitement." *Journal of Experimental Psychology: General* 143 (3): 1144–58.

Brown, D. W., R. F. Anda, H. Tiemeier, V. J. Felitti, V. J. Edwards, J. B. Croft, and W. H. Giles. 2009. "Adverse Childhood Experiences and the Risk of Premature Mortality." *American Journal of Preventive Medicine* 37: 389–96.

Casey, C. Y., M. A. Greenberg, P. M. Nicassio, R. E. Harpin, and D. Hubbard. 2008. "Transition from Acute to Chronic Pain and Disability: A Model Including Cognitive, Affective, and Trauma Factors." *Pain* 134: 69–79.

Chiesa, A., and A. Serretti. 2009. "Mindfulness-Based Stress Reduction for Stress Management in Healthy People: A Review and Meta-analysis." *Journal of Alternative and Complementary Medicine* 15 (5): 593–600.

Cohen, S., T. Kamarck, and R. Mermelstein. 1983. "A Global Measure of Perceived Stress." *Journal of Health and Social Behavior* 24: 385–96.

Cohen, S., D. A. J. Tyrrell, and A. P. Smith. 1991. "Psychological Stress and Susceptibility to the Common Cold." *New England Journal of Medicine* 325: 606–12.

Cohen, S., and T. A. Wills. 1985. "Stress, Social Support, and the Buffering Hypothesis." *Psychological Bulletin* 98: 310–57.

Cole, S. W., L. C. Hawkley, J. M. Arevalo, C. Y. Sung, R. M. Rose, and J. T. Cacioppo. 2007. "Social Regulation of Gene Expression in Human Leukocytes." *Genome Biology* 8 (9): R189.

Crum, A. J., P. Salovey, and S. Achor. 2013. "Rethinking Stress: The Role of Mindsets in Determining the Stress Response." *Journal of Personality and Social Psychology* 104: 716–33.

Cryder, C. E., S. Springer, and C. K. Morewedge. 2012. "Guilty Feelings, Targeted Actions." *Personality and Social Psychology Bulletin* 38: 607–18.

Curtis, R., A. Groarke, and F. Sullivan. 2014. "Stress and Self-Efficacy Predict Psychological Adjustment at Diagnosis of Prostate Cancer." *Scientific Reports* 4: 5569.

Davidson, R., J. D. Kabat-Zinn, M. Schumacher, D. Rosenkranz, S. F. Muller, F. Santorelli, A. Urbanowski, K. Harrington, K. Bonus, and J. F. Sheridan. 2003. "Alterations in Brain and Immune Function Produced by Mindfulness Meditation." *Psychosomatic Medicine* 65: 564–70.

Davis, C., S. Nolen-Hoeksema, and J. Larson. 1998. "Making Sense of Loss and Benefiting from the Experience: Two Construals of Meaning." *Journal of Personality and Social Psychology* 75: 561–74.

Davis, C. G., C. B. Wortman, D. R. Lehman, and R. C. Silver. 2000. "Searching for Meaning in Loss: Are Clinical Assumptions Correct?" *Death Studies* 24: 497–540.

Dienstbier, R. A. 1989. "Arousal and Physiological Toughness: Implications for Mental and Physical Health." *Psychological Review* 96 (1): 84–100.

Duckworth, A. 2016. *Grit: The Power of Passion and Perseverance.* New York: Scribner.

Duckworth, A. L., C. Peterson, M. D. Matthews, and D. R. Kelly. 2007. "Grit: Perseverance and Passion for Long-Term Goals." *Journal of Personality and Social Psychology* 92 (6): 1087–1101.

Duhigg, C. 2012. *The Power of Habit: Why We Do What We Do in Life and Business.* New York: Random House.

Emmons, R. A., and M. E. McCullough. 2003. "Counting Blessings vs. Burdens: An Experimental Investigation of Gratitude and Subjective Well-Being in Daily Life." *Journal of Personality and Social Psychology* 84: 377–89.

Epel, E. S., E. H. Blackburn, J. Lin, F. S. Dhabhar, N. E. Adler, J. D. Morrow, and R. M. Cawthon. 2004. "Accelerated Telomere Shortening in Response to Life Stress." *Proceedings of the National Academy of Sciences* 101 (41): 17312–15.

Epel, E. S., B. McEwen, T. Seeman, K. Matthews, G. Castellazzo, K. D. Brownell, J. Bell, and J. R. Ickovics. 2000. "Stress and Body Shape: Stress-Induced Cortisol Secretion Is Consistently Greater Among Women with Central Fat." *Psychosomatic Medicine* 62 (5): 623–32.

Eskreis-Winkler, L., E. Shulman, S. Beal, and A. L. Duckworth. 2014. "The Grit Effect: Predicting Retention in the Military, the Workplace, School and Marriage." *Frontiers in Personality Science and Individual Differences* 5 (36): 1–12.

Felitti, V. J., R. F. Anda, D. Nordenberg, D. F. Williamson, A. M. Spitz, V. Edwards, M. P. Koss, and J. S. Marks. 1998. "Relationship of Childhood Abuse and Household Dysfunction to Many of the Leading Causes of Death in Adults. The Adverse Childhood Experiences (ACE) Study." *American Journal of Preventive Medicine* 14: 245–58.

Flett, G. L., P. L. Hewitt, and M. Heisel. 2014. "The Destructiveness of Perfectionism Revisited: Implications for the Assessment of Suicide Risk and the Prevention of Suicide." *Review of General Psychology* 18 (3): 156–72.

Fox, K. C., S. Nijeboer, M. L. Dixon, J. L. Floman, M. Ellamil, S. P. Rumak, P. Sedlmeier, and K. Christoff. 2014. "Is Meditation Associated with Altered Brain Structure? A Systematic Review and Meta-Analysis of Morphometric Neuroimaging in Meditation Practitioners." *Neuroscience Biobehavioral Reviews* 43: 48–73.

Frattaroli, J. 2006. "Experimental Disclosure and Its Moderators: A Meta-Analysis." *Psychological Bulletin* 132: 823–65.

Fredrickson, B. L. 2004. "The Broaden-and-Build Theory of Positive Emotions." *Philosophical Transactions of the Royal Society B: Biological Sciences* 359: 1367–78.

Fredrickson, B. L., and T. Joiner. 2002. "Positive Emotions Trigger Upward Spirals Toward Emotional Well-Being." *Psychological Science* 13: 172–75.

Fredrickson, B. L., R. A. Mancuso, C. Branigan, and M. M. Tugade. 2000. "The Undoing Effect of Positive Emotions." *Motivation and Emotion* 24 (4): 237–58.

Germer, C. K. 2009. *The Mindful Path to Self-Compassion: Freeing Yourself from Destructive Thoughts and Emotions.* New York: Guilford Press.

Gilbert, P. 2010. *The Compassionate Mind: A New Approach to Life's Challenges.* Oakland, CA: New Harbinger Publications.

Glaser, R., and J. K. Kiecolt-Glaser. 2005. "Stress-Induced Immune Dysfunction: Implications for Health." *Nature Reviews Immunology* 5 (3): 243–51.

Glaser, R., G. R. Pearson, R. H. Bonneau, B. A. Esterling, C. Atkinson, J. K. Kiecolt-Glaser. 1993. "Stress and the Memory T-Cell Response to the Epstein-Barr Virus in Healthy Medical Students." *Health Psychology* 12 (6): 435–42.

Gross, J. J., and R. A. Thompson. 2007. "Emotion Regulation: Conceptual Foundations." In *Handbook of Emotion Regulation,* edited by James J. Gross. New York: Guilford Press.

Grossman, P., L. Niemann, S. Schmidt, and H. Walach. 2003. "Mindfulness-Based Stress Reduction and Health Benefits: A Meta-analysis." *Focus on Alternative and Complementary Therapies* 8 (4): 500.

Gunnar, M. R., K. Frenn, S. S. Wewerka, and M. J. van Ryzin. 2009. "Moderate vs. Severe Early Life Stress: Associations with Stress Reactivity and Regulation in 10–12-Year-Old Children." *Psychoneuroendocrinology* 34: 62–75.

Hanson, R. 2009. *Buddha's Brain: The Practical Neuroscience of Happiness, Love, and Wisdom.* With R. Mendius. Oakland, CA: New Harbinger Publications.

Hölzel, B. K., J. Carmody, M. Vangel, C. Congleton, S. M. Yerramsetti, T. Gard, and S. W. Lazar. 2011. "Mindfulness Practice Leads to Increases in Regional Brain Gray Matter Density." *Psychiatry Research: Neuroimaging* 191 (1): 36–43.

Hommel, K. A., J. L. Wagner, J. M. Chaney, and L. L. Mullins. 2001. "Prospective Contributions of Attributional Style and Arthritis Helplessness to Disability in Rheumatoid Arthritis." *International Journal of Behavioral Medicine* 8 (3): 208–19.

Kabat-Zinn, J. 1982. "An Out-Patient Program in Behavioral Medicine for Chronic Pain Patients Based on the Practice of Mindfulness Meditation: Theoretical Considerations and Preliminary Results." *General Hospital Psychiatry* 4: 33–47.

———. 1994. *Wherever You Go, There You Are: Mindfulness Meditation in Everyday Life.* New York: Hyperion.

Kabat-Zinn, J., L. Lipworth, and R. Burney. 1985. "The Clinical Use of Mindfulness Meditation for the Self-Regulation of Chronic Pain." *Journal of Behavioral Medicine* 8: 163–90.

Kalm, L. M., and R. D. Semba. 2005. "They Starved so that Others Be Better Fed: Remembering Ancel Keys and the Minnesota Experiment." *Journal of Nutrition* 135 (6): 1347–52.

Keyes, K. M., M. L. Hatzenbuehler., B. F. Grant, and D. S. Hasin. 2012. "Stress and Alcohol: Epidemiologic Evidence." *Alcohol Research: Current Reviews* 34 (4): 391–400.

Khoury, B., T. Lecomte, G. Fortin, M. Masse, P. Therien, V. Bouchard, M. Chapleau, K. Paquin, and S. G. Hofmann. 2013. "Mindfulness-Based Therapy: A Comprehensive Meta-analysis." *Clinical Psychology Review* 33 (6): 763–71.

Kobasa, S. C. 1979. "Stressful Life Events, Personality, and Health: An Inquiry into Hardiness." *Journal of Personality and Social Psychology* 37: 1–11.

Kornfield, J. 1993. *A Path with Heart: A Guide Through the Perils and Promises of Spiritual Life.* New York: Bantam Books.

Kripke, D. L., L. Garfinkel, D. L. Wingard, M. R. Klauber, and M. R. Marler. 2002. "Mortality Associated with Sleep Duration and Insomnia." *Archives of General Psychiatry* 59: 131–36.

Langer, E., and J. Rodin. 1976. "The Effects of Choice and Enhanced Personal Responsibility for the Aged: A Field Experiment in an Institutional Setting." *Journal of Personality and Social Psychology* 19: 191–98.

Lepore, S. J., and M. A. Greenberg. 2002. "Mending Broken Hearts: Effects of Expressive Writing on Mood, Cognitive Processing, Social Adjustment and Health Following a Relationship Breakup." *Psychology and Health* 17: 547–60.

Loprinzi, P. D., and B. J. Cardinal. 2011. "Association Between Objectively-Measured Physical Activity and Sleep, NHANES 2005–2006." *Mental Health and Physical Activity* 4 (2): 65–69.

Lutz, A., L. L. Greischar, N. B. Rawlings, M. Ricard, and R. J. Davidson. 2004. "Long-Term Meditators Self-Induce High-Amplitude Gamma Synchrony During Mental Practice." *Proceedings of the National Academy of Science* 101: 16369–73.

Lutz, J., U. Herwig, S. Opialla, A. Hittmeyer, L. Jäncke, M. Rufer, M. Grosse Holtforth, and A. B. Brühl. 2014. "Mindfulness and Emotion Regulation—an fMRI Study." *Social Cognitive and Affective Neuroscience* 9 (6): 776–85.

MacBeth, A., and A. Gumley. 2012. "Exploring Compassion: A Meta-analysis of the Association Between Self-Compassion and Psychopathology." *Clinical Psychology Review* 32 (6): 545–52.

Marmot, M. G., G. Davey Smith, S. Stansfeld, C. Patel, F. North, J. Head, I. White, E. Brunner, and A. Feeney. 1991. "Health Inequalities Among British Civil Servants: The Whitehall II Study." *Lancet* 337 (8754): 1387–93.

Masten, A. S., and M. J. Reed. 2002. "Resilience in Development." In *Handbook of Positive Psychology*, edited by C. R. Snyder and S. Lopez. New York: Oxford University Press.

McEwen, B. S. 1998. "Protective and Damaging Effects of Stress Mediators." *New England Journal of Medicine* 338: 171–79.

McGonigal, K. 2015. *The Upside of Stress: Why Stress Is Good for You and How to Get Good at It.* New York: Penguin.

McKee-Ryan, F., Song, Z., Wanberg, C. R., and Kinicki, A. J. 2005. *Psychological and Physical Well-Being During Unemployment: A Meta-Analytic Study. Journal of Applied Psychology* 90 (1): 53–76.

Mineka, S., M. Gunnar, and M. Champoux. 1986. "Control and Early Socioemotional Development: Infant Rhesus Monkeys Reared in Controllable vs. Uncontrollable Environments." *Child Development* 57: 1241–56.

Mineka, S., and J. F. Kihlstrom. 1978. "Unpredictable and Uncontrollable Events: A New Perspective on Experimental Neurosis." *Journal of Abnormal Psychology* 87 (2): 256–71.

Moyer, C. A., M. P. Donnelly, J. C. Anderson, K. C. Valek, S. J. Huckaby, D. A. Wiederholt, R. L. Doty, A. S. Rehlinger, and B. L. Rice. 2011. "Frontal Electroencephalographic Asymmetry Associated with Positive Emotion Is Produced by Very Brief Meditation Training." *Psychological Science* 22, 1277–79.

Mullainathan, S., and E. Shafir. 2013. *Scarcity: The New Science of Having Less and How It Defines Our Lives.* New York: Picador, Reprint Edition.

Neff, K. D. 2011. *Self-Compassion: The Proven Power of Being Kind to Yourself.* New York: William Morrow.

Neff, K. D., Y. Hsieh, and K. Dejitterat. 2005. "Self-Compassion, Achievement Goals, and Coping with Academic Failure." *Self and Identity* 4: 263–87.

Neff, K. D., K. Kirkpatrick, and S. S. Rude. 2007. "Self-Compassion and Its Link to Adaptive Psychological Functioning." *Journal of Research in Personality* 41: 139–54.

Neff, K. D., and R. Vonk. 2009. "Self-Compassion vs. Global Self-Esteem: Two Different Ways of Relating to Oneself." *Journal of Personality* 77: 23–50.

Neupert, S. D., D. M. Almeida, and S. T. Charles. 2007. "Age Differences in Reactivity to Daily Stressors: The Role of Personal Control." *Journal of Gerontology, Series B: Psychological and Social Sciences* 62: 216–25.

Nolen-Hoeksema, S. 2000. "The Role of Rumination in Depressive Disorders and Mixed Anxiety/Depressive Symptoms." *Journal of Abnormal Psychology* 109: 504–11.

Nolen-Hoeksema, S., and C. G. Davis. 1999. "'Thanks for Sharing That: Ruminators and Their Social Support Networks." *Journal of Personality and Social Psychology* 77: 801–14.

Palomino, R. A., P. M. Nicassio, M. A. Greenberg, and E. P. Medina. 2007. "Helplessness and Loss as Mediators Between Pain and Depressive Symptoms in Fibromyalgia." *Pain* 129: 185–94.

Pagliari, R., and L. Peyrin. 1995. "Norepinephrine Release in the Rat Frontal Cortex Under Treadmill Exercise: A Study with Microdialysis." *Journal of Applied Physiology* 78: 2121–30.

Pennebaker, J. W., and C. K. Chung. 2011. "Expressive Writing: Connections to Physical and Mental Health." In *The Oxford Handbook of Health Psychology*, edited by Howard S. Friedman. Oxford: Oxford University Press.

Puterman, E., J. Lin, E. Blackburn, A. O'Donovan, N. Adler, and E. Epel. 2010. "The Power of Exercise: Buffering the Effect of Chronic Stress on Telomere Length." *PLoS One* 5 (5): e10837.

Rhodes, A. M. 2015. "Claiming Peaceful Embodiment Through Yoga in the Aftermath of Trauma." *Complementary Therapies in Clinical Practice* 21: 247–56.

Rodin, J. 1986. "Aging and Health: Effects of the Sense of Control." *Science* 233: 1271–76.

Rodin, J., and E. J. Langer. 1977. "Long-Term Effects of a Control-Relevant Intervention with the Institutionalized Aged." *Journal of Personality and Social Psychology* 35 (12): 897–902.

Rosengren, A., K. Orth-Gomér, H. Wedel, and L. Wilhelmsen. 1993. "Stressful Life Events, Social Support, and Mortality in Men Born in 1933." *British Medical Journal* 307 (6912): 1102–5.

Rutter, M. 2006. "Implications of Resilience Concepts for Scientific Understanding." *Annals of the New York Academy of Sciences* 1094: 1–12.

Salzberg, S. 2002. *Lovingkindness: The Revolutionary Art of Happiness.* Rev. ed. Boston: Shambhala.

Sapolsky, R. M. 2004. *Why Zebras Don't Get Ulcers.* New York: Times Books.

Sbarra, D. A., H. L. Smith, and R. M. Mehl. 2012. "When Leaving Your Ex, Love Yourself: Observational Ratings of Self-Compassion Predict the Course of Emotional Recovery Following Marital Separation." *Psychological Science* 23 (3): 261–69.

Seehagen, S., S. Schneider, J. Rudolph, S. Ernst, and N. Zmyj. 2015. "Stress Impairs Cognitive Flexibility in Infants." *Proceedings of the National Academy of Science* 112 (41): 12882–86.

Seery, M. D., E. A. Holman, and R. C. Silver. 2010. "Whatever Does Not Kill Us: Cumulative Lifetime Adversity, Vulnerability, and Resilience." *Journal of Personality and Social Psychology* 99: 1025–41.

Seery, M. D. 2011. "Resilience: A Silver Lining to Experiencing Adverse Life Events?" *Current Directions in Psychological Science* 20: 390–94.

Segerstrom, S. C., S. E. Taylor, M. E. Kemeny, and J. L. Fahey. 1998. "Optimism Is Associated with Mood, Coping, and Immune Change in Response to Stress." *Journal of Personality and Social Psychology* 74: 1646–55.

Seligman, M. E. P., and S. F. Maier. 1967. "Failure to Escape Traumatic Shock." *Journal of Experimental Psychology* 74 (1): 1–9.

Shah, A., S. Mullainathan, and E. Shafir. 2012. "Some Consequences of Having Too Little." *Science* 338: 682–85.

Siegel, D. J. 2010. *Mindsight: The New Science of Personal Transformation.* New York: Bantam.

Siegle, G. J., R. E. Ingram, and G. E. Matt. 2002. "Affective Interference: Explanation for Negative Information Processing Biases in Dysphoria?" *Cognitive Therapy and Research* 26: 73–88.

Smyth, J., A. Stone, A. Hurewitz, and A. Kaell. 1999. "Effects of Writing About Stressful Experiences on Symptom Reduction in

Patients with Asthma or Rheumatoid Arthritis: A Randomized Trial." *Journal of the American Medical Association* 281: 1304–9.

Spera, S. P., E. D. Buhrfeind, and J. W. Pennebaker. 1994. "Expressive Writing and Coping with Job Loss." *Academy of Management Journal.* 37: 722–33.

Stahl, B., and E. Goldstein. 2010. *A Mindfulness-Based Stress Reduction Workbook*. Oakland, CA: New Harbinger Publications.

Stanton, A. L., S. Danoff-Burg, L. A. Sworowski, C. A. Collins, A. Branstetter, A. Rodriguez-Hanley, S. B. Kirk, and J. L. Austenfeld. 2002. "Randomized, Controlled Trial of Written Emotional Expression and Benefit Finding in Breast Cancer Patients." *Journal of Clinical Oncology* 20: 4160–68.

Stein, N., S. Folkman, T. Trabasso, and T. A. Richards. 1997. "Appraisal and Goal Processes as Predictors of Psychological Well-Being in Bereaved Caregivers." *Journal of Personality and Social Psychology* 72: 872–84.

Teegarden, S. L., and T. L. Bale. 2008. "Effects of Stress on Dietary Preference and Intake Are Dependent on Access and Stress Sensitivity." *Physiology and Behavior* 93: 713–23.

Thompson, S. C., A. Sobolew-Shubin, M. E. Galbraith, L. Schwankovsky, and D. Cruzen. 1993. "Maintaining Perceptions of Control: Finding Perceived Control in Low-Control Circumstances." *Journal of Personality and Social Psychology* 64 (2): 293–304.

Tolle, E. 2004. *The Power of Now: A Guide to Spiritual Enlightenment*. Novato, CA: New World Library.

Troxel, W. M., K. A. Matthews, L. C. Gallo, and L. H. Kuller. 2005. "Marital Quality and Occurrence of the Metabolic Syndrome in Women." *Archives of Internal Medicine* 165 (9): 1022–27.

Tugade, M. M., and B. L. Fredrickson. 2004. "Resilient Individuals Use Positive Emotions to Bounce Back from Negative Emotional Experiences." *Journal of Personality and Social Psychology* 86 (2): 320–33.

Van den Berg, M., J. Maas, R. Muller, A. Braun, W. Kaandorp, R. van Lien, M. N. van Poppel, W. van Mechelen, and A. E. van den Berg. 2015. "Autonomic Nervous System Responses to Viewing Green and Built Settings: Differentiating Between Sympathetic and Parasympathetic Activity." *International Journal of Environmental Research and Public Health* 12: 15860–74.

Wallston, K. A., B. S. Wallston, S. Smith, and C. Dobbins. 1987. "Perceived Control and Health." *Current Psychological Research and Reviews* 6: 5–25.

Wegner, D. M., R. Erber, and S. Zanakos. 1993. "Ironic Processes in the Mental Control of Mood and Mood-Related Thought." *Journal of Personality and Social Psychology* 65: 1093–1104.

Wegner, D., D. Schneider, S. Carter, and T. White. 1987. "Paradoxical Effects of Thought Suppression." *Journal of Personality and Social Psychology* 53 (1): 5–13.

Weiss, J. M., H. I. Glazer, L. A. Pohorecky, J. Brick, and N. E. Miller. 1975. "Effects of Chronic Exposure to Stressors on Avoidance-Escape Behavior and on Brain Norepinephrine." *Psychosomatic Medicine* 37: 522–34.

Weiss, J. M., E. A. Stone, and N. Harrell. 1970. "Coping Behavior and Brain Norepinephrine Level in Rats." *Journal of Comparative and Physiological Psychology* 72 (1): 153–60.

Werner, E. E., and R. S. Smith. 2001. *Journeys from Childhood to Midlife: Risk, Resilience, and Recovery.* New York: Cornell University Press.

Wren, A. A., T. J. Somers, M. A. Wright, M. C. Goetz, M. R. Leary, A. M. Fras, B. K. Huh, and L. L. Rogers. 2012. "Self-Compassion in Patients with Persistent Musculoskeletal Pain: Relationship of Self-Compassion to Adjustment to Persistent Pain." *Journal of Pain and Symptom Management* 43 (4): 759–70.

Young, J. E., J. S. Klosko, and M. Weishaar. 2003. *Schema Therapy: A Practitioner's Guide.* New York: Guilford Press.

Zawadzki, M. J., J. E. Graham, and W. Gerin. 2013. "Rumination and Anxiety Mediate the Effect of Loneliness on Depressed Mood and Poor Sleep Quality in College Students." *Health Psychology* 32: 212–22.

Melanie Greenberg, PhD, is a practicing psychologist and executive coach in Marin County, CA, and an expert on managing stress, health, and relationships using proven techniques from neuroscience, mindfulness, and cognitive behavioral therapy (CBT). With more than twenty years of experience as a professor, writer, researcher, clinician, and coach, Greenberg has delivered workshops and talks to national and international audiences. She writes the *Mindful Self-Express* blog for *Psychology Today,* and is a popular media expert who has been quoted on cnn.com, forbes.com, BBC Radio, ABC News, *Yahoo! Shine,* and *Lifehacker,* as well as in *Self, Redbook, Men's Health, Women's Health, Fitness Magazine, Women's Day, Cosmopolitan,* and *The Huffington Post.* She has also appeared on radio shows like *Leading With Emotional Intelligence, The Best People We Know, Inner Healers,* and *Winning Life Through Pain.* Greenberg was named one of the 30 Most Prominent Psychologists to Follow on Twitter.

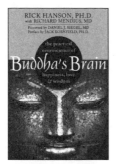
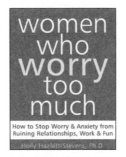
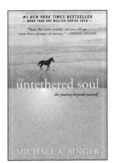
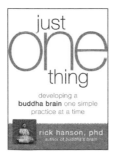
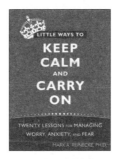
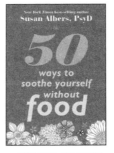
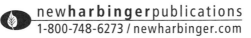 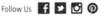

Register your **new harbinger** titles for additional benefits!

When you register your **new harbinger** title—purchased in any format, from any source—you get access to benefits like the following:

- Downloadable accessories like printable worksheets and extra content

- Instructional videos and audio files

- Information about updates, corrections, and new editions

Not every title has accessories, but we're adding new material all the time.

Access free accessories in 3 easy steps:

1. Sign in at NewHarbinger.com (or **register** to create an account).

2. Click on **register a book**. Search for your title and click the **register** button when it appears.

3. Click on the **book cover or title** to go to its details page. Click on **accessories** to view and access files.

That's all there is to it!

If you need help, visit:

NewHarbinger.com/accessories

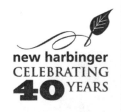

new harbinger
CELEBRATING
40 YEARS